3

MRCOG II
Short Essay Questions

D1584669

This book is dedicated to our families:
to Tanweer, Sofia and Shafiq Abedin;
and to Zena, Omar and Abdallah Sharif

MRCOG II
Short Essay Questions

Parveen Abedin MRCOG
Specialist Registrar in Obstetrics and Gynaecology
Birmingham Women's Hospital
Birmingham, UK

Khaldoun W. Sharif MD, MRCOG, MFFP
Consultant Obstetrician and Gynaecologist
Director of Assisted Conception Services
RCOG District Tutor
Birmingham Women's Hospital;
Honorary Senior Lecturer in Obstetrics and Gynaecology
The University of Birmingham
Birmingham, UK

ABGDIN

WQ 18 H0302815

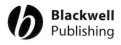

Blackwell
Publishing

© 2003 by Blackwell Publishing Ltd
Blackwell Publishing, Inc., 350 Main Street, Malden, Massachusetts 02148–5018, USA
Blackwell Publishing Ltd, 9600 Garsington Road, Oxford OX4 2DQ, UK
Blackwell Publishing Asia Pty Ltd, 550 Swanston Street, Carlton South, Victoria 3053, Australia
Blackwell Verlag GmbH, Kurfürstendamm 57, 10707 Berlin, Germany

First published 2003 by Blackwell Publishing Ltd

Library of Congress Cataloging-in-Publication Data
Abedin, Parveen.
    MRCOG II : short essay questions/by Parveen Abedin,
Khaldoun W. Sharif.
        p. ; cm.
    ISBN 1-40510-020-6
1. Obstetrics—Examinations, questions, etc. 2. Gynecology—Examinations, questions, etc.
I. Sharif, Khaldoun W. II. Title. III. Title: MRCOG 2. IV. Title: MRCOG two.
    [DNLM: 1. Genital Diseases, Female—Examination Questions. 2. Gynecology—Examination
Questions. 3. Obstetrics—Examination Questions. 4. Pregnancy Complications—Examination
Questions. WP 18.2 A138m 2003]

RG111   . A345 2003
618'.076—dc21

                                                                          2002013167

ISBN 1-4051-0020-6

A catalogue record for this title is available from the British Library

Set in 9.5/12pt Minion by Kolam Information Services Pvt. Ltd, Pondicherry, India
Printed and bound in Great Britain by TJ International, Padstow, UK

Commissioning Editor: Stuart Taylor
Editorial Assistant: Heather Johnston
Production Editor: Rebecca Huxley
Production Controller: Chris Downs

For further information on Blackwell Publishing, visit our website:
www.blackwell-science.com

Contents

Preface

Obtaining the Membership of the Royal College of Obstetricians and Gynaecologists (MRCOG) is an essential step to becoming a specialist in obstetrics and gynaecology in the United Kingdom (UK) as well as many other countries. The Part 2 MRCOG Examination has changed considerably in recent years, almost beyond recognition. Perhaps the most significant change is the introduction of the short-answer essay papers. These form two-thirds of the Part 2 written examination, which each candidate has to pass before being allowed to sit the oral assessment examination. Therefore, the short-answer essay papers effectively hold the key to the MRCOG. In fact, in recent examinations, poor performance in the short-answer essay papers has been identified by the RCOG as the most common cause of failure; only 20% of candidates on average manage to pass the written examination! This book has been written to address this issue. It provides advice on how to prepare for, and answer examination essays. It also contains 154 examination-like essays, together with notes on their model answers. These essays are divided into the recognized branches and sub-specialities of obstetrics and gynaecology to aid both practice and revision.

The advice and examples given in this book are born out of our experience in training our junior colleagues and running MRCOG courses over a number of years. In all our teaching we emphasize that knowledge and training could be obtained from many sources. However, as all experienced doctors know, the most informative teachers are the patients, to whom we dedicate this book.

P.A.
K.W.S.
Birmingham, 2003

Acknowledgements

We wish to thank Dr Imogen Morgan, Consultant Neonatologist, and Dr Bolarinda Ola, Research Fellow at the Birmingham Women's Hospital for providing invaluable contributions to particular chapters in areas of their expertise.

How to use this book

We believe that if you fully understand the examination system, the different types of essay questions asked, and how to prepare for and answer each type you are far more likely to pass. Therefore, to get the maximum benefit from this book, we strongly recommend that you first read the following chapter before you attempt any of the essays. Most candidates are often eager to attempt essays rather than read advice, but this is rather like starting an unfamiliar journey without planning your path. One can easily get lost.

When you come to attempt the examples in the book, you are advised to do so under examination-like conditions. You should try to answer 5 essays in 2 hours. Running out of time is a common problem in the examination, and practice makes perfect.

Having written your answers, you should get them assessed by someone who is experienced and familiar with the examination system. The hospital hierarchical system ensures many such doctors are available. In addition, the notes on model answers provided in this book will tell you what points should be included in your answer. The notes and the assessment are complementary.

The Part 2 MRCOG short-answer essay questions

Introduction

The written examination in the Part 2 MRCOG contains two essay papers. The first paper, lasting 2 h, consists of five short-answer essay questions primarily concerning obstetrics and those relevant aspects of medicine, surgery, paediatrics and gynaecology. The second paper, also lasting 2 h, consists of five short-answer essay questions primarily concerning gynaecology and those relevant aspects of medicine, surgery and obstetrics.

Importance of the essays

The essay papers are the most important part of the Part 2 MRCOG examination. They form two-thirds of the written examination (MCQ being the remaining third). Only candidates who pass the written can proceed to the oral assessment examination. A poor performance in the essays cannot be compensated for by a good performance in the MCQ and will most probably result in failure in the written paper and, consequently, in the whole examination. Indeed, the RCOG has repeatedly identified this as a problem area and the main cause of failure in the Part 2 examination (about 80% of candidates in recent examination diets have failed in the written papers). The importance of adequate preparation for the essays cannot be overemphasized.

What is being assessed by the essay papers

A number of differing qualities are being assessed at the same time. These include:
- *Factual knowledge*: this is the basis for all your answers in the examination. This knowledge, however, is not only gained from reading textbooks and journals, but also from clinical practice. Remember, the MRCOG is a clinical examination aimed at obstetric and gynaecological Specialist Registrars (SpR/years 1–3) in the UK and their equivalents. Therefore, the knowledge expected from you at the examination is similar to what you are expected to know as an SpR.

Having said that, it is worth noting that poor knowledge is rarely the cause of poor performance in the essays. This is not to say that knowledge is not necessary, but rather not enough.

- *Analysis and solution of specific problems*: totally factual knowledge that could be tested with simple yes/no options is assessed using MCQ. The essays assess controversial issues that require providing a carefully considered opinion on a given scenario. This requires breaking down the problem into its basic components, then allotting sensible priorities to each component. This can equally apply to clinical scenarios (e.g. shoulder dystocia) or organizational issues (e.g. early pregnancy assessment units). The emphasis here is as much on knowing what to do as it is on knowing why you are doing it. Simple enumeration or listing is not adequate, and these are common causes of poor performance in the essays. Also, remember it is a clinical examination, and a clinical approach in your analysis is required.
- *Communication*: no matter how up-to-date and comprehensive your factual knowledge is, or how brilliant you are in analytical thinking, you cannot pass the examination if you do not communicate well in writing. This requires you to be proficient in the use of *basic* English (grammar, syntax and punctuation). Also your handwriting should be legible, as examiners cannot mark what they cannot read.
- *The ability to answer the question*: a common cause of failure is not answering the question. This usually results from not understanding the question.
- *Time management*: the fact that you have to answer the questions in a limited time (five questions in 2 h) is one of the most stressful aspects of the examination. Time management is essential. In the examination (and during practice) allocate 20–24 min to each question and decide what to include and what to omit from the answer. Each question has equal marks allocated to it, and a good performance in a particular question can rarely compensate for a very poor performance in another.

Adequate Preparation

Practice makes perfect, and it is even more important with this type of 'short-answer' essays currently used in the MRCOG. Most candidates associate essay questions with spending about an hour writing many pages in the answer. This was correct with the previously used 'long-answer' essay questions. The current examination system, however, allows only about 24 min for each answer and requires no more than two sides of A4 paper. Prior practice is essential here to be able to concentrate your thoughts and write down the relevant points in this relatively limited time and space.

The Questions

There are various types of essay questions that could be asked in the MRCOG. Admittedly, questions usually come in a 'combination' form between the different types. Here, however, we will discuss each type individually for the purpose of illustration.

1 The first type is the 'Discuss/Critically evaluate/Critically appraise/Compare and contrast/Debate...' question. Examples are:

- *Discuss the use of anticoagulant drugs in obstetrics.*
- *Hysterectomy for dysfunctional uterine bleeding is out of date. Discuss.*
- *Critically appraise the use of the colposcope in gynaecological practice.*

When answering this type of question, you should imagine that you are the learned expert giving a lecture to post-Membership doctors or writing an editorial about the subject in a medical journal. In fact, editorials and commentaries in journals are very good illustrations of how these questions should be answered. They start by briefly outlining the condition and its importance (e.g. incidence, effect on maternal/perinatal mortality/morbidity). They then go on to dedicate the main bulk of the essay to presenting a critical account of the predisposing factors, aetiology, presentation, symptoms, signs, special investigations, differential diagnosis, prevention, treatment, follow-up and so on as appropriate. Controversial issues are explored in depth, and the pros and cons of different options are discussed before reaching a reasoned conclusion.

2 The second type is the 'clinical situation' essay. Theoretically it is the easiest to answer as it asks candidates to write about what they do in everyday clinical practice. Examples include:

- *A 19-year-old-woman attends the gynaecological clinic because she has not menstruated for 1 year. Discuss your management.*
- *Describe the management of a woman with infertility and oligomenorrhoea.*
- *Discuss the management of a patient with fulminating pre-eclampsia.*

The best way to answer this type of question is to reflect on your clinical practice and write what you would do, and why, if confronted with such a clinical situation. This will almost always be in the format of presentation, history, examination, investigations, treatment and follow-up.

3 The third type is by far the commonest type that appears in the MRCOG. It is a combination of the first two types, in the sense that it requires critical evaluation of your management of a particular scenario.

This should not be difficult for a well-practised clinician like you. For every patient you actually see in real life you have to define the problem (or problems), the aims of your management, how best to achieve these aims (given the available situation and resources) and the reasons behind your choices. This last point brings in the issues of alternatives, other options, pros, cons, and—not least—patient's choices and values.

Does this sound like a formidable task? Well, it shouldn't be, because you have been doing it for a number of years: seeing patients and managing them competently. Probably the part some doctors have not been doing so well is thinking why they have been doing a particular thing or choosing a certain option. Start from this moment thinking (and finding out) why you are doing what you are doing with every patient. By the time you reach the examination, this type of question will become much easier. Better still, work will become more enjoyable and effective.

Examples of these questions include:

- *A woman presents with a third-trimester stillbirth. She does not consent to postmortem examination of the baby. Justify the steps of your investigations.*
- *A 31-year-old woman has unexplained infertility of 2 years' duration. Compare and contrast the management options.*

4 This type of question also asks you to write about something you have been doing all the time: telling patients about their problem, what it means to them, what you are going to do about it, and why. These 'counselling' questions do fit better in the 'Oral Assessment' part of the examination, but they frequently appear in the essays. Doctors are repeatedly asked to explain to patients *in writing* about their illnesses (e.g. leaflets, the Internet), and this type of question assesses your ability in doing so. Counselling her means assisting the patient to make a choice or decision, by discussing the options and relating them to her particular situation.

Examples of these questions include:

- *A 45-year-old woman is going to have a hysterectomy for heavy periods. How would you counsel her about removing her ovaries?*
- *An 18-year-old woman in her first pregnancy is booking at 16 weeks. She requests an ultrasound scan to 'check that all is well with the baby'. How would you counsel her?*

The Answer

In the examination you are given an answer booklet, with *only* two sides of lined A4 available for the answer of each essay. You will also be given coloured paper for rough notes. The examiners will not see these.

Read the question TWICE

This is the commonest advice given in any examination. Yet, it is the least followed. The number of MRCOG candidates who misread words like 'infertility' as 'fertility', 'pre-eclampsia' as 'eclampsia' or write extensively about the past obstetric history in answering a question about a primigravida makes repeating this advice very valid. Please, read the question TWICE.

Underline the key words

After reading the question twice, underline the *key* words. These will tell you what type of question it is, what exactly it is asking for, and in what particular situation or context. You should look for these elements in every essay question. If you get any of them wrong, you will simply not be answering the question. The key words will tell you what the question wants and, as importantly, what it does not want. Writing what is not required attracts no marks, wastes valuable time, and gives a bad impression to the examiner.

The following example should illustrate these points:

1 Discuss the use of anticoagulant drugs in obstetrics.
   The three key points are:

- *Discuss* (a critical evaluation-type question).
- *Use* (all uses—prophylaxis, treatment, DVT, PE, recurrent pregnancy loss with antiphospholipid).
- *Anticoagulant drugs* (main subject, include all drugs—heparin, warfarin, aspirin, etc.).
- *Obstetrics* (not gynaecology).

Anatomy of the essay
Plan

This is the vertebral column of the answer on which you can attach other parts and build a complete essay. Having read the question TWICE, underlined the key words and understood what is required, you should now spend about 2 min planning the general structure of the answer. The skill is in deciding the most important points to include *before* you start writing down the answer. This is particularly important because you have a relatively short time to answer each question (average 24 min). If you do not plan your answer in advance, you may spend a long time discussing an important point, only to discover that there is another equally important point that deserves discussion, but with no time available. The instructions to examiners indicate specific marks for each point, and elaboration on one point will not compensate for omission of another. Although the plan is not written down on the answer sheet and is not marked, nevertheless, it helps you to organize your thoughts and makes essay writing a straightforward process. In the examination the plan should be written on the coloured rough paper provided and not in the answer book. For example, if you are asked to discuss an operation it will be easier (for both you and the examiner) if your discussion is planned broadly into three parts: preoperative, intraoperative and postoperative care. Other examples that may be of use to you in the essay planning include:

- Preconception. Antenatal (1st, 2nd, 3rd trimesters). Intrapartum. Postnatal.
- History. Examination. Investigations. Treatment. Follow-up. Rehabilitation/Home care.
- Effect of pregnancy on the disease. Effect of the disease on pregnancy (mother, fetus, neonate, breast feeding, contraception).
- Causes: obstetric/non-obstetric. Maternal/fetal. Congenital/acquired. Gynaecological/non-gynaecological. Other 'issues' that are useful in various situations include:
- Senior involvement.
- Multidisciplinary approach.
- Team approach.
- Social support.
- Timing and mode of delivery.
- Home care.
- Involvement of partner/family.

The introduction
This is the first brief paragraph of the 'Discuss/Evaluate/Critically appraise/Debate' type of essays, where you give a broad overview of the subject and what you intend to discuss in the main body. You also show the examiner that you understand the importance of the subject in question. This should be in the form of factual information. For example, when answering a question about thromboembolism or anticoagulant drugs, it is very pertinent to introduce your essay by mentioning that thromboembolism is one of the commonest causes of maternal mortality in the UK. Similarly, in answering a question about infertility you should mention that it affects 1 in 6 couples. Percentages and figures are the most powerful tools for illustrating factual information, and you are well advised to learn those related to common conditions. Important points include effects on peri-

natal/maternal mortality/morbidity, incidence, 5-year survival rates and cost-effectiveness.

Also in the other types of questions that deal with a particular case scenario the introduction is important. Here you start by stating what your aims are in brief. For example in questions about counselling you can introduce the answers by stating that your aim is to assist the patient in making a decision about, say, prophylactic oophorectomy by providing her with easily understood information about the options and their implications. Another example is in a question about the management of a case of eclampsia. You can introduce your answer by stating your aims (provide basic life support, control fits, prevent recurrence, control blood pressure, assess the situation both maternal and fetal, stabilize the condition, and delivery). You can see that a well-written introduction will not only impress your examiner but also assist you in writing the rest of the answer.

Body of the essay

This consists of a number of paragraphs, each discussing a distinct issue related to the subject. Emphasis on the discussion is very important, as at the Membership level simple listing and enumeration is neither adequate nor acceptable. What is required is a mature discussion reflecting your understanding of the controversial issues and leading to a reasoned conclusion. If dealing with a clinical situation, please remember that the sequences of your actions as well as the reasons behind them are very important.

If you have written a logical well thought out plan you should have no trouble in writing this part of the answer. The plan will tell you what other important issues you need to discuss so you do not 'over do it' with a particular issue at the expense of others. It will also provide you with the 'filing compartments' you need to fill so you are less likely to forget important items.

The conclusion

This is the final paragraph in the essay and the part the examiner reads last before deciding your mark. Therefore, it should be positively strong. A good essay which ends abruptly without a conclusion (most probably because the candidate has run out of time) is unlikely to attract high marks.

It is all too easy to fall into the trap of repetition when writing the conclusion. If all it does is just repeat what you have already said in the rest of the essay then it is probably a waste of effort and time. Ideally, it should be an opportunity to pick out the most significant parts from the answer and comment on their practical implications, prognosis, or future development—as appropriate.

Reviewing the answer

Again this is vital advice that is rarely followed. You should allow a couple of minutes to review your answer at the end. You WILL find mistakes and you should correct them in a tidy way (see below). Correcting your mistakes tells the examiner that not only can you recognize your mistakes but are prepared to correct them—as all safe doctors should be.

Handwriting and presentation

It is a myth that good doctors have bad handwriting. They may have started with bad handwriting, as they have started with not knowing how to do operations, but with practice and persistence they should become good at both.

It goes without saying that the examiners cannot mark what they cannot read. It is of primary importance that you should write legibly. Many people think that they can never improve their handwriting, but this is not true. Legible handwriting is a skill, not a talent, and it is learned by practice. Practice makes perfect, or at least makes legible. You need to practice writing larger, clearly and slowly. Some suggest writing with a 'fluid-ink' pen, as this will make you write slowly. You have to make sure, however, that you do not smudge the ink on the paper, which is easily done with these pens. The best advice is to try different types of pens during your practice until you find the one that suits you most and makes your writing clearer.

You also have to make sure that your answer is tidy, with not much crossing out. If you make a mistake, it is better to use a single line to cross it, as this will appear more tidy than using multiple heavy lines. The best thing, of course, is to avoid crossing out altogether.

A good tip, next to being perfect and making no mistakes, is to use correction fluid (e.g. Tipp-Ex) to cover any mistake. Several brands are available in the market, and you are well advised to try some of them during your practice and decide on the most appropriate one to take to the examination.

To aid the clarity of the answer, it is worth writing headings for the main paragraphs and sparingly underlining the key words using a different colour (e.g. red). Do remember to take a ruler to the examination, as zigzag lines are not very presentable.

Timing the answer

One of the main aspects of examinations in general is the limited time available for answering. In the Part 2 written examination you are given 2 h to answer five essay questions, and you should dedicate about 20–25 min for each question. Many candidates, having found that they know more about one or more questions than the rest (which is not unusual), spend most of the time answering those questions at the expense of the others. This is based on the mistaken belief that an excellent answer will compensate for a very poor one.

The first 2 min should be dedicated to the plan, the following 20 min to the actual essay, and the last 2 min to revision and corrections. This revision is very important as the absence or presence of small words like 'not' can make a big difference to the meaning. What you can write in 20 min, you can say in 3–4 min depending on your speed. It might appear unfair that you are expected to write an essay about a big subject like preterm labour in such a short space of time. It is the purpose of the examination, however, to test your ability in presenting the important and relevant information in the allocated time.

Good basic English

Your aim is to convey your scientific thoughts clearly and concisely using good English language. This is best achieved by dividing your essay into paragraphs each addressing a separate issue. Short sentences, each containing no more than two clauses and presenting a single clear idea are easier to construct and understand than complex multiclaused sentences. Thoughts should flow logically and effortlessly from one sentence to the next.

The rules of good basic English should be adhered to. These include grammar (the relation between words) and syntax (the construction of sentences).

Examiners' Instructions

For each essay, the examiners are given a structured marking scheme with suggested guidelines on how many marks to be allocated to each part of the answer. Half marks may be used for components within the answers but the total must be rounded *down* to a whole mark. There is an ongoing debate between examiners on how many marks to allocate for logical coherent expression and overall impression. What is not debatable, however, is that a good answer always attracts high marks.

Section A:
Obstetrics

Chapter 1
Fetomaternal medicine

Chapter 1: Questions

Answers are on pp. 18–54

Q1. A 24-year-old woman intending to become pregnant comes to you for advice. She is fit and healthy with no major medical problems or adverse family history. What advice would you impart to her?

Q2. Justify the use of a booking ultrasound scan at the first antenatal visit to the hospital?

Q3. Critically appraise the screening methods for Down's syndrome in the first and second trimester.

Q4. A 32-year-old primigravida attends the antenatal booking clinic at 9 weeks. She weighs 130 kg and has a body mass index of 39.6 but has no relevant medical history or other risk factors. How would you modify her antenatal and intrapartum care in view of her obesity?

Q5. A woman comes to you at 10 weeks in her fourth pregnancy having had three previous mid-trimester abortions. A recurrent miscarriage screen done earlier has not shown up any abnormalities. Justify your management of this pregnancy.

Q6. A 45-year-old woman is referred by her GP in her first pregnancy. She is 8 weeks pregnant. How will you modify her care in view of her age?

Q7. A 14-year-old girl books with you in her first pregnancy at 16 weeks. Critically appraise the management of her pregnancy.

Q8. A woman with a known history of chronic hypertension books at 11 weeks gestation in her first pregnancy. Her booking blood pressure is 140/95 mmHg. Justify the principles of management of her pregnancy.

Q9. A woman presents to you at 37 weeks in her first pregnancy with a frank breech presentation. You counsel her with a view to a caesarean section but she refuses, saying that she would only consider this as a last resort. How will you go about managing this case?

Q10. Critically appraise the contraindications to external cephalic version.

Q11. A patient is referred to you at 23 weeks into her third pregnancy with anti-c antibody titres of 25 iu/L. Her past obstetric history includes an intrauterine fetal death at 26 weeks due to hydrops fetalis. How do you propose to manage the rest of her pregnancy?

Q12. A woman at 34 weeks gestation in her first pregnancy is found to have polyhydramnios. Critically appraise your management.

Q13. A woman turns up to the antenatal clinic in your hospital for the first time. She is unbooked and by dates is around 26 weeks pregnant. She admits to smoking heroin with a history of injecting it in the past. How will you go about managing her pregnancy?

Q14. While eliciting a booking history from a nulliparous woman at 9 weeks gestation, she tells you she is a heavy smoker. Critically appraise the advice you would give her regarding this.

Q15. A 30-year-old woman books at 8 weeks gestation in her second pregnancy. Her first child is in care due to social problems. She is an alcoholic. Critically appraise your management of her pregnancy.

Q16. A woman attending a routine antenatal clinic inquires about epidural analgesia in labour. Unfortunately an anaesthetist cannot be found to answer her questions. Describe briefly how you would counsel the woman.

Q17. A woman is referred to the antenatal clinic in her third pregnancy. Her previous obstetric history includes two preterm deliveries at 32 and 30 weeks, respectively. Critically appraise your management of her pregnancy.

Q18. A woman booking in her first pregnancy is found to have a platelet count of 100×10^9/L. This falls as the pregnancy advances until at 30 weeks it is down to 50×10^9/L. Justify your management.

Q19. A routine full blood count in a pregnant woman taken at her booking visit reveals a haemoglobin of 7 g/dL, with the following red cell indices: MCV 96 fl, MCH 27 pg, MCHC 30 g/dL. Critically appraise your management.

Q20. A woman has a booking scan which reveals a monochorionic twin gestation. How will you plan the management of her pregnancy? A scan at 26 weeks reveals an increased amniotic fluid index in twin one and a decreased amniotic fluid index in twin two. How will you manage the rest of her pregnancy?

Q21. You are a registrar on labour ward and are called to see a lady in labour. She is at term and is expecting twins with the first twin cephalic. She then proceeds to labour and delivers the first twin uneventfully. Examination then reveals that the second twin is a transverse lie with intact membranes. How will you proceed with the rest of her labour?

Q22. A routine mid-trimester scan on a woman reveals an anterior abdominal wall defect, in the form of an exomphalos. The couple are very worried and come to you for counselling and further management of the pregnancy. Justify your approach to this case.

Q23. Critically appraise the management of a pregnancy where a left-sided congenital diaphragmatic hernia has been diagnosed on ultrasound scan at 16 weeks.

Q24. A 26-year-old 16-week pregnant woman is found to have a fetal choroid plexus cyst on the booking scan. Justify your management, relevant to this finding.

Q25. A couple present to the antenatal clinic after a mid-trimester scan which has revealed ventriculomegaly. How will you counsel the couple and manage the pregnancy?

Q26. A woman is referred to you by her community midwife at 28 weeks gestation with a symphysiofundal height of 22 cm. Critically appraise your management.

Q27. A woman presents to delivery suite with premature contractions at 23 weeks gestation. A vaginal examination reveals her cervix to be 5 cm dilated with intact membranes. Critically appraise the steps you will take to manage the case.

Q28. A woman books at 9 weeks in her second pregnancy, having had a caesarean section in her previous pregnancy. Critically appraise how you will decide on the mode of delivery.

Q29. Evaluate how you could reduce the morbidity and mortality associated with caesarean sections.

Q30. Critically appraise the surgical techniques which may improve the outcome of caesarean sections.

Q31. You are the registrar on call for labour ward and are called to see a patient in labour by her midwife. She is primiparous at term, and has progressed from 7 cm to 10 cm cervical dilatation in 5 h. She has been pushing for an hour and a half without success. Critically appraise your management.

Q32. A woman in her first pregnancy is seen in the antenatal clinic at 41 weeks, having had no previous problems in the pregnancy. Outline your plan of management and justify the steps you would take.

Q33. Clinical risk management is becoming more and more important in the practice of obstetrics. Justify this statement and explain how you would ensure risk management in your unit.

Q34. A couple with a 2-year-old child with cerebral palsy come to you to find out if the management of the labour could have been responsible for the condition. They vaguely recollect an abnormal cardiotocograph in labour, which led to an emergency caesarean section. Their child was on the neonatal intensive care unit for a few weeks. Critically appraise the steps you will take to counsel the couple.

Q35. A woman complains of severe dyspareunia at a routine 6-week postnatal appointment following a normal vaginal delivery. Justify your investigations and management.

Q36. A woman in her second pregnancy comes to you wanting to know about the potential risks and benefits of collecting cord blood for banking of haemopoietic stem cells (HSC) at the time of delivery. She has a healthy 3-year-old child and there is no history of any genetic or acquired diseases in the family. How will you counsel her?

Q37. Discuss the specific factors to be taken into consideration when planning an elective caesarean section at 39 weeks in a patient with an anterior placenta praevia, who has had two previous caesarean sections.

Q38. Critically discuss the value of urine testing in pregnancy.

Q39. Critically discuss the drugs used for thromboprophylaxis in obstetric practice.

Q40. A pregnant woman at 10 weeks gestation had been in contact with a child who developed chickenpox 2 days later. Justify your advice and management.

Chapter 1: **Answers**

Q1. A 24-year-old woman intending to become pregnant comes to you for advice. She is fit and healthy with no major medical problems or adverse family history. What advice would you impart to her?

A1.

- In the prepregnancy clinic it is important to stratify patients into high, moderate or low risk categories based on general health and the presence of medical conditions, previous obstetric history and any significant family history, especially of genetic disorders.
- In the above case, there are no mitigating factors present and thus the patient can be safely assigned to the low risk group and thus can be reassured.
- It is important to impart correct prepregnancy advice to her. This includes advice on prepregnancy weight, with the BMI ideally being between 20 and 25.
- Periconceptual folic acid should be prescribed, which is 400 µg daily to be taken around 12 weeks before conception to around 13 weeks gestation.
- Alcohol and smoking should ideally be stopped or reduced while pregnant as they can both cause low birth weight. Alcohol, depending upon amount consumed, can cause alcohol-related birth defects (ARBD), as well as neurological impairment and the fetal alcohol syndrome.
- Vegans should be advised to have additional iron and vitamin supplements, with ethnic groups lacking exposure to sunlight being advised on the consumption of extra vitamin D.
- It is imperative to check prepregnancy rubella status with non-immune women receiving immunization and being advised not to become pregnant for at least 12 weeks afterwards.

Q2. Justify the use of a booking ultrasound scan at the first antenatal visit to the hospital?

A2.

- The advantages of scanning all pregnant women at their first antenatal visit to hospital has to be balanced against the considerable cost it entails to the already beleaguered health service.
- A booking scan in early pregnancy ensures viability of the pregnancy.
- A booking scan in the first trimester can accurately date the pregnancy. This is important for good antenatal care. Dating can be achieved with great accuracy when the pregnancy is less than 24 weeks. Accurate knowledge of dates will enhance the accuracy of serum screening programmes.

Randomized studies suggest that the induction rate may be reduced by nearly 40% in pregnancies in which gestational age is known.

- An early scan can identify multiple pregnancies and also determine chorionicity. This is best undertaken at less than 14 weeks. In the case of monochorionic pregnancies, closer monitoring of the pregnancy may enable the earlier detection of complications such as twin-to-twin transfusion and this may in turn determine a better outcome for the pregnancy.
- Nuchal translucency measurements are undertaken at the early scan. This is used to modify the age-related risk of trisomy 21. It has also been shown to be associated with other abnormal outcomes such as cardiac defects, trisomies 18 and 13 and Turner's syndrome.
- Cervical length can be assessed on the early scan. Measurement of cervical length and the shape of the internal os may be looked for to indicate the competence of the cervix. This information may be useful in women with a history of recurrent mid-trimester pregnancy losses in deciding the feasibility of inserting a cervical suture.
- Gross structural anomalies such as anencephaly can be detected at the time of an initial scan though caution must be exercised in diagnosing major fetal anomalies any time in the first trimester.
- Maternal structures can also be evaluated in the first trimester. This includes ovarian cysts, fibroids, etc.

Q3. Critically appraise the screening methods for Down's syndrome in the first and second trimester.

A3.

- The aim of screening tests is to give an estimate of high risk of having an affected pregnancy, so that further invasive diagnostic testing can be undertaken in these women to confirm whether the condition is present.
- Serum screening methods in the second trimester focus on the estimation of certain markers, which may be raised or lowered in affected pregnancies. The 'double test', which combines advanced maternal age with estimation of hCG and α-fetoprotein levels in maternal serum have a detection rate of 60% for a false positive rate of 5%. The 'triple test' adds the estimation of unconjugated oestriol, which raises the detection rate to 68% with a similar false positive rate. The addition of serum inhibin A, the 'quadruple test', reaches a sensitivity of 76%.
- It is important to bear in mind that serum marker concentrations are affected by factors such as maternal weight, being inversely proportional, recent bleeding, which increases the serum α-fetoprotein levels, and the

presence of insulin-dependent diabetes mellitus. They are also unreliable in multiple gestations, and require accurate ultrasound assessment of gestational age.

- Approximately one-third of Down's syndrome fetuses have associated structural abnormalities which may be detected on ultrasound scans. These include congenital heart defects, duodenal atresia, cystic hygromas, exomphalos and ventriculomegaly. However, the detection of these structural defects results in the detection of only 33% of Down's syndrome fetuses. There are certain soft tissue markers associated with the condition, which are better at picking up affected pregnancies. The presence of one or more markers in a high risk population has a sensitivity of 87% with a false positive rate of 6%. The best combination of soft tissue markers are nuchal fold thickness, short humerus and renal pyelectasis.

- Free β-hCG and pregnancy-associated plasma protein A (PAPP-A), are the two biochemical markers which are increased in the first trimester in affected pregnancies. Screening programmes combining advanced maternal age with these two markers in the first trimester will detect 60–68% of Down's syndrome fetuses with a false positive rate of <5%. The sensitivities of this screening method are inferior however, in clinical practice, to current second-trimester screening.

- In high risk populations, where investigations are being carried out for advanced maternal age, nuchal translucency thickness measurements in the first trimester detect 77% of Down's syndrome pregnancies with a false positive rate of 5%. This is comparable to serum screening in the second trimester, with the advantages of early detection which allow for earlier invasive diagnostic testing such as chorionic villus biopsy, with a subsequent earlier and less traumatizing termination of pregnancy. The disadvantages are the high operator dependence for accurate measurements, difficulties in reproducibility of measurements, along with the earlier detection of pregnancies which may have been fated to miscarry anyway. Added to this is the higher risk of miscarriage with earlier invasive tests such as chorionic villus biopsy (2% compared to 1% for amniocentesis in the second trimester).

- The combination of first-trimester biochemical markers and nuchal translucency detection on ultrasound reaches sensitivities of 90% for a false positive rate of 5%. This is thus much higher than second-trimester screening methods.

- Integrated screening, which involves combining screening in both the first and second trimesters, reaches detection rates of 94% with a false positive rate of 5%. This includes first trimester nuchal translucency and PAPP-A measurements, with second trimester α-fetoprotein, serum oestriol and hCG measurements, which may be favoured by older women wishing to obtain as much information as possible before undergoing invasive diagnostic testing with all the inherent risks involved.

- It is important that the woman involved is given accurate information and is made to understand the implications before opting into such a screening programme.

Q4. A 32-year-old primigravida attends the antenatal booking clinic at 9 weeks. She weighs 130 kg and has a body mass index of 39.6 but has no relevant medical history or other risk factors. How would you modify her antenatal and intrapartum care in view of her obesity?

A4.

- In a pregnant obese patient it is important to identify the particular risks involved and the potential problems that may arise in their management. First and foremost it may be difficult to establish viability and dating of the pregnancy without transvaginal scanning. They are more at risk of developing pregnancy-induced hypertension, gestational diabetes and thromboembolic phenomenon.
- Dietary advice is appropriate and these patients should be referred to a dietitian. However, weight loss in pregnancy should be discouraged. A glucose tolerance test should be considered and careful monitoring of blood pressure with an appropriate sized cuff should be undertaken. Clinical abdominal examinations may be unhelpful, thus necessitating serial scans for growth.
- Electronic fetal monitoring with an abdominal transducer may not be feasible and a fetal scalp electrode may have to be used. There is a risk of shoulder dystocia and thus senior medical and midwifery staff should be available at delivery. Caesarean sections are more hazardous both surgically and anaesthetically and again senior staff should be involved. Thromboprophylaxis is mandatory in the event of a caesarean section and must be considered in vaginal, especially instrumental deliveries.

Q5. A woman comes to you at 10 weeks in her fourth pregnancy having had three previous mid-trimester abortions. A recurrent miscarriage screen done earlier has not shown up any abnormalities. Justify your management of this pregnancy.

A5.

- In such a case, it is important to go into a detailed history of the miscarriages, including any signs of chorioamnionitis, and the history of onset of labour with the typical features of painless dilatation of the cervix pointing to a diagnosis of cervical incompetence. The results of any postmortem examinations should be gone into if available.

- In case cervical incompetence is suspected, serial ultrasound scans should be undertaken to look for cervical length and any signs of funneling of the cervix. If this is found to be the case, better pregnancy outcomes have been shown by the MRC/RCOG trial in certain cases which undergo cervical cerclage procedures. These can be in the form of a vaginal suture, either a McDonald's or Shirodkar's suture. They are usually undertaken electively at around 14 weeks. In the former, a purse string of a non-absorbable suture material such as mersilene is inserted around the cervix at the cervicovaginal junction. The latter involves an incision in the supravaginal portion of the cervix to expose and reflect the bladder so that a non-absorbable suture such as mersilene can be placed higher around the cervix than is possible with a McDonald's suture.
- Alternatively, a transabdominal suture can be used though this is usually confined to those cases in which vaginal sutures have failed. This involves a low transverse abdominal incision with the incision of the peritoneum and reflection of the bladder. A mersilene tape is then inserted at the level of the internal os and tied posteriorly. Removal of a vaginal suture is undertaken routinely at 37–38 weeks or sooner if the patient threatens to miscarry or go into preterm labour. Abdominal sutures are usually left in place with delivery being affected by an elective caesarean section. The suture can be removed after the woman's family is complete.
- The pregnancy should be carefully monitored with routine screens for vaginal infection and to look for onset of preterm labour. Any infections should be aggressively treated with antibiotics. It is important to offer the couple psychological support through the pregnancy because of the bad obstetric history and to deal with them in a sympathetic manner. They should have ready access to the hospital and specialist care in the case of any problems.

Q6. A 45-year-old woman is referred by her GP in her first pregnancy. She is 8 weeks pregnant. How will you modify her care in view of her age?
A6.
- The main problems associated with advanced maternal age in the first pregnancy are a higher rate of miscarriage, chromosomal abnormalities, multiple gestation, hypertensive disorders, uterine fibroids, gestational diabetes, prolonged labour, higher rates of operative delivery, bleeding disorders including placenta praevia, low birth weight and increased

perinatal mortality. All these points must be borne in mind while planning her antenatal and intrapartum care.

- The woman should be carefully counselled about the risk of aneuploidy (trisomy 21, 18, 13, sex chromosome aberrations) at this age, which is around 1 in 20–30. Karyotyping in the form of chorionic villus biopsy or amniocentesis should be offered to her with the understanding that though CVS will obtain a quicker result and thus an opportunity for an earlier termination (around 14–15 weeks), there is a higher risk of miscarriage (1 in 50 as compared to 1 in 100 for amniocentesis).
- Careful antenatal follow-up to monitor fetal and maternal condition is mandatory. This includes regular blood pressure and urine monitoring, serial scans for growth if clinical suspicion of intrauterine growth retardation, and placental site localization.
- There is a higher risk of dystocia and it is recommended that these women are delivered in a specialist unit. Close monitoring of the fetal condition during labour, especially the second stage, is recommended.

Q7. A 14-year-old girl books with you in her first pregnancy at 16 weeks. Critically appraise the management of her pregnancy.

A7.

- Teenage pregnancies are associated with social, rather than physical or medical problems.
- It is important to be aware that cigarette smoking, alcohol consumption and illicit drug abuse are all common amongst pregnant adolescents with all the associated problems.
- These girls are particularly at risk of nutritional deficiencies and sexually transmitted diseases.
- Medical complications include anaemia, urinary tract infections, hypertension, preterm labour and low birth weight, higher analgesia requirement, and operative assistance during labour, short interval to the next pregnancy and sudden infant death syndrome.
- As compliance with antenatal care tends to be poor, it is important to do early scans to confirm gestational age. Identification of other risk factors is also important.
- Social support should be offered in close collaboration with the family doctor, an empathetic midwife, and a social worker.
- Continuous support during labour by the mother's partner or family members should be encouraged.

Social
Medi
Iuteap
SIDS .

- In exceptionally young adolescents, confinement in a specialist unit is advisable in view of obstructed labour due to the small size of the immature pelvis.

Q8. A woman with a known history of chronic hypertension books at 11 weeks gestation in her first pregnancy. Her booking blood pressure is 140/95 mmHg. Justify the principles of management of her pregnancy.

A8.

- The incidence of chronic hypertension in pregnancy is around 0.5–3%. Essential hypertension is responsible for 90% of this. The rest are due to secondary hypertension. These can be secondary to renal disease, endocrine disorders such as diabetes with vascular involvement, thyrotoxicosis or rarely phaeochromocytoma, or due to collagen vascular disease such as systemic lupus erythematosus.
- In cases of mild chronic hypertension the incidence of perinatal mortality and morbidity and that of maternal morbidity is not increased from the general population.
- In cases of severe hypertension with blood pressure at or above 160/110 mmHg, there are considerable risks involved. These are mainly that of superimposed pre-eclampsia, which may occur in 25–50% of cases. Other risks are that of congestive cardiac failure, intracerebral haemorrhage, acute renal failure and placental abruption.
- During the initial visit, a detailed evaluation of the aetiology and severity of the hypertension should be made. Laboratory investigations should include urine analysis and culture, electrolytes, uric acid, blood sugar, and a 24-h urine collection for protein and creatinine clearance. Patients with severe hypertension or proteinuria in the first trimester should undergo a chest X-ray, ECG, antinuclear antibody tests, and should be tested for the presence of lupus anticoagulant and anticardiolipin antibodies.
- Women with mild hypertension can have their antihypertensive medication discontinued at their booking visit. Careful monitoring should then ensue. Only half will need subsequent medication. Patients should be taken off antihypertensive medication with potential adverse effects on the fetus such as angiotensin-converting enzyme inhibitors and diuretics.
- Antihypertensive therapy should be started when the diastolic blood pressure reaches 110 mmHg. This is to prevent cerebrovascular accidents. Methyldopa, is a good first-line antihypertensive agent, with labetalol being a good second-line agent.

- Careful fetal monitoring, with serial growth scans should be undertaken. The pregnancy may be continued till term, unless superimposed pre-eclampsia or fetal growth restriction supervenes.
- The care of women with severe superimposed pre-eclampsia should be undertaken in a fetal medicine unit in a tertiary referral centre with appropriate liaison with specialists such as nephrologists.
- Though chronic hypertension *per se* is not a cause for concern, it becomes one when complications such as pre-eclampsia supervene. This necessitates a very careful monitoring of maternal and fetal condition and consideration of early delivery in these cases.

Q9. A woman presents to you at 37 weeks in her first pregnancy with a frank breech presentation. You counsel her with a view to a caesarean section but she refuses, saying that she would only consider this as a last resort. How will you go about managing this case?

A9.

- The breech presentation at term has always posed a challenge to the clinicians managing the pregnancy. A recently concluded multicentre randomized trial has confirmed that vaginal delivery is more hazardous to the term breech than elective caesarean section, with the overall risk of perinatal death reduced by 75% in the latter case. However, if in spite of proper counselling the woman refuses to be delivered by caesarean section, it is important to respect her wishes and ensure that every possible step is taken to ensure the best possible outcome.
- External cephalic version should be offered as a means to correct the presentation to cephalic. In experienced hands, this offers a reduction of over 80% in the odds of a non-cephalic birth, with a reduction in caesarean section rate of 50%.
- ECV should be carried out at term, preferably on a labour ward with facilities available for emergency delivery if required. Cardiotocography should be performed, with ultrasound guidance being found helpful.
- Tocolysis is helpful in ensuring a successful outcome in ECV.
- In case of failure of ECV, the woman should again be fully counselled regarding the pros and cons of a vaginal breech delivery vs. a caesarean section. If she still insists on a trial of vaginal delivery, it should be ensured that a sufficiently experienced obstetrician is available to conduct the delivery.
- X-ray pelvimetry has not been shown to be helpful in predicting outcome.

- It is essential to carefully monitor the progress of labour as well as fetal well-being. Fetal blood sampling from the buttocks provides an accurate estimation of acid–base status.
- There is no evidence that epidural analgesia is required and in selected cases induction or augmentation can be done.
- It is important at all times to ensure that the woman is fully aware of all interventions undertaken with full documentation by all concerned medical staff.
- In such a case where the woman with a term breech presentation refuses to undergo a caesarean section, the most important things to ensure is the involvement of senior obstetric staff at an early stage, with proper counselling and the offer of alternative options. The conduct of the delivery should again be handled by staff experienced in delivering breech babies, with continuous monitoring to ensure fetal well-being.

Q10. Critically appraise the contraindications to external cephalic version.

A10.

- External cephalic version is the process of external abdominal manipulation to convert the presentation of the fetus to a cephalic one.
- In present practice, it is most commonly used to convert a breech presentation to a cephalic one. It should not be carried out prior to 37 weeks as this may give rise to preterm labour, or may necessitate the delivery of a premature baby were a complication to supervene.
- Contraindications to ECV in the mother include, low lying placenta, or where there is a known cause for the abnormal presentation such as cervical or uterine fibroids or a bicornuate or subseptate uterus.
- Previous caesarean sections are not an absolute contraindication, though it should not be attempted with classical uterine scars because of the greater risk of rupture before the onset of labour.
- Severe pregnancy-induced hypertension, pre-eclampsia and antepartum haemorrhage are also contraindications. Though the procedure can be attempted in women with spontaneous rupture of membranes, the success rate is considerably lower because of the reduced liquor.
- It should not be carried out unless all procedures are in place to effect an immediate delivery in case of complications. Undue force should not be used, and the patient should not be sedated or anaesthetized. Cardiotocographic monitoring should be done before and immediately following the procedure to ensure fetal well-being.

- Contraindications in the fetus include fetal compromise in the form of intrauterine growth restriction, oligohydramnios, or fetal anaemia due to isoimmunization. Neurological abnormalities in the fetus may cause reduced movements and breech presentation, thus it is important to carry out a scan for growth, liquor volume and biophysical profiles to ensure fetal well-being prior to attempting the procedure.
- Before the procedure, the couple should be counselled about the methods and the risks involved. They may opt not to have it done in which case their wishes will have to be respected.

Q11. A patient is referred to you at 23 weeks into her third pregnancy with anti-c antibody titres of 25 iu/L. Her past obstetric history includes an intrauterine fetal death at 26 weeks due to hydrops fetalis. How do you propose to manage the rest of her pregnancy?

A11.

- Fetal haemolytic disease due to maternal alloimmunization remains a serious and common cause of perinatal mortality and morbidity throughout the world. Due to widespread immunoprophylaxis in rhesus negative women, the importance of anti-D antigen in causing alloimmunization is diminishing and hence the importance of other antigens such as anti-c are increasing, with up to 50% of cases in the western world being reported due to them.
- It is important that all cases of maternal alloimmunization with the potential for serious consequences for the fetus be treated in a referral centre with experience in dealing with such cases and the back up of expert neonatal care and blood transfusion services if necessary. Thus cases care from hospitals not used to dealing with them should be appropriately referred to the nearest tertiary referral centre.
- Fetal sequelae of haemolytic disease relate to the development of severe fetal anaemia. These should be looked for on high resolution ultrasonography. Ascites and pericardial effusions with an increase in cardiac biventicular diameter along with high peak flow Doppler velocities in the middle cerebral artery are indicative of fetal anaemia.
- In this particular case, with a history of sensitization in a former pregnancy and with serum antibody levels which are apparently above the critical laboratory titre to cause potential problems, some form of invasive testing to determine whether the fetus is being affected, should be undertaken. The two tests usually undertaken include either amniocentesis or cordocentesis.

- Amniocentesis is done to obtain amniotic fluid which is then subjected to spectrophotometry and the value is plotted onto the 'modified Liley's curve'. Depending upon where the value falls on the curve, a decision for fetal therapy is made. The polymerase chain reaction (PCR) can be used to determine whether the fetus is antigen positive or not.
- The disadvantages with amniocentesis are the risks of enhanced maternal sensitization, amnionitis, rupture of membranes and the fact that this is an indirect test for fetal anaemia. However, depending on the facilities available and the physician's experience it may be the only appropriate test.
- Fetal blood sampling via cordocentesis is associated with a slightly higher fetal loss rate but is a more direct test for fetal anaemia with a zero false positive rate.
- Fetal blood transfusions are carried out when the fetal haematocrit falls below 30%. They are usually intravascular or more rarely, intraperitoneal.
- The transfusion may need to be repeated depending on the decline of the fetal haematocrit and signs of fetal hydrops on serial scanning.
- In non-transfused fetuses, delivery is usually planned between 37 and 38 weeks. There are no contraindications to vaginal delivery unless other obstetric indications supervene.
- Delivery in transfused fetuses or in those showing persistent signs of hydrops is usually planned earlier, with the administration of steroids for lung maturity if this is planned earlier than 36 weeks.
- Neonatologists should be involved from the beginning, as neonatal double volume exchange transfusion or phototherapy may be needed due to hyperbilirubinaemia.

Q12. A woman at 34 weeks gestation in her first pregnancy is found to have polyhydramnios. Critically appraise your management.
A12.
- Polyhydramnios is defined as an amniotic fluid index more than the 95th percentile for gestational age.
- Polyhydramnios can be due to maternal diabetes mellitus, impairment of fetal swallowing as in anencephaly and chromosomal abnormalities, duodenal atresia or viral infections. Idiopathic polyhydramnios, where no cause is identified, occurs in a large percentage of cases.
- It is important to take a complete history, including that of diabetes mellitus, and perform a high resolution ultrasound to detect the degree of polyhydramnios, detailed anomaly scan to look for abnormalities of the fetal gastrointestinal system and central nervous system, and to do a

GI
CNS
Intns.

fetal viral screen for TORCH and parvovirus. Karyotyping may be recommended if indicated.

- Idiopathic polyhydramnios even in structurally normal fetuses is associated with a higher perinatal mortality and morbidity rate due to its association with⌠preterm rupture of membranes, preterm delivery, unstable lie, cord prolapse and placental abruption due to uterine distension⌡
- ⌠Management is aimed at relieving maternal symptoms and preventing preterm labour.⌡Mild asymptomatic polyhydramnios is managed expectantly. In moderate to severe polyhydramnios which is giving rise to excessive maternal symptoms several options are available. Amnioreduction, where transabdominal aspiration of fluid is done under ultrasound control is one option and it can prolong gestation by preventing preterm labour. Other options are the administration of prostaglandin inhibitors such as indomethacin. The drawback of this is its association with premature closure of the ductus, cerebral vasoconstriction and impaired renal function.
- Polyhydramnios *per se* if not associated with other anomalies is not a cause for concern unless it becomes severe and starts giving rise to maternal symptoms. These women should be kept a close eye on and monitored for symptoms of preterm labour.

Q13. A woman turns up to the antenatal clinic in your hospital for the first time. She is unbooked and by dates is around 26 weeks pregnant. She admits to smoking heroin with a history of injecting it in the past. How will you go about managing her pregnancy?

A13.
- The most important aspect of taking care of a drug addict in pregnancy is a non-judgemental approach to her care with the involvement of a multidisciplinary team consisting of an obstetrician, midwives, addiction counsellors, social workers, neonatologists, health visitors and family doctors.
- A detailed history and clinical examination should be undertaken including the types and quantities of drugs ingested and the nutritional status of the mother with additional confounding factors such as smoking and alcohol being kept in mind.
- Booking bloods should be undertaken with testing for hepatitis B and C virus and HIV testing.
- It is important to stress the risks of heroin addiction for the baby, including the particular risks of street heroin with its unreliability in

strength, which produces uncontrolled levels. She should be strongly encouraged to go onto a detoxification programme with maintenance therapy with methadone. The dose is maintained as long as required and later in the pregnancy, if the woman is agreeable, it can be slowly reduced.

- A scan at the first visit is undertaken to confirm gestation and subsequently, she should have serial scans every 2 weeks to monitor growth. Umbilical artery Doppler studies and liquor assessment is undertaken weekly from 34 weeks. There is an association with intrauterine growth restriction, preterm labour and premature delivery.
- A meeting is usually held around 32 weeks gestation with the woman and her partner present along with the drug team, health visitor and social worker to decide the needs of the mother and baby and the necessity for a prenatal child protection conference.
- There may be problems with analgesic requirements during labour because of the need for higher doses of opiates. Epidural analgesia may thus be a good idea.
- The infant is monitored for neonatal narcotic abstinence syndrome (NAS) which is characterized by hyperirritability, jitteriness, a high pitched cry and poor feeding.
- Drug addiction in pregnant women is a problem that should be dealt with by a multiprofessional team who not only take care of the woman during her pregnancy but also ensure that she is followed up postnatally and that the welfare of the child is ensured.

Q14. While eliciting a booking history from a nulliparous woman at 9 weeks gestation, she tells you she is a heavy smoker. Critically appraise the advice you would give her regarding this.

A14.

- Smoking is one of the few potentially preventable factors associated with low birth weight babies and perinatal death. It is important to counsel women properly about the risks of smoking in pregnancy.
- Mothers who smoke in pregnancy generally deliver babies weighing 100–300 g less than children born to non-smokers. This is directly proportional to the number of cigarettes smoked.
- Premature delivery is twice as common in smokers. Smoking also increases the likelihood of loss of a fetus from 28 weeks gestation up to the first seven days of life, with low Apgar scores and an association with acidosis in the neonate.

- There is a significant increase in the risk of placental abruption, placenta praevia, bleeding in early and late pregnancy, and preterm premature rupture of membranes in smokers.
- Sudden infant death syndrome (SIDS) is much commoner in infants of smoking mothers, with an average of 27% of deaths attributed to SIDS.
- There is a strong relationship between increased maternal mortality from conditions such as placenta praevia and placental abruption.

Q15. A 30-year-old woman books at 8 weeks gestation in her second pregnancy. Her first child is in care due to social problems. She is an alcoholic. Critically appraise your management of her pregnancy.

A15.

- In order to diagnose the problem, the 'TACE' questionnaire is used. In this, four questions are put to the woman: (1) How many drinks does it take to make you feel high? (tolerance) (2) Have people annoyed you by criticizing your drinking? (3) Have you ever felt you should cut down? (4) Do you need a drink first thing in the morning (eye opener)? A score of two or more points is considered diagnostic of heavy drinking.
- It is important to take a detailed history, and calculate the amount of alcohol consumed, as this has a direct bearing on fetal outcome and degree of neurological impairment. No adverse effects on pregnancy outcome have been proven with a consumption of less than 120 g of alcohol per week (15 units). Reduction in birth weight is associated with consumption of more than 120 g per week. More than 160 g (20 units) is associated with intellectual impairment.
- Fetal alcohol syndrome is a rare event, with an incidence of 1.5–3.5 per 1000 live births. It includes fetal growth retardation, central nervous system involvement and characteristic facial dysmorphology.
- These women are poor antenatal clinic attenders and therefore must be followed up by health personnel in the community.
- They are often lacking in a nutritious diet, which compounds the effects of the alcohol on the pregnancy. Proper dietary advice is thus essential.
- Regular review with growth scans is mandatory.
- There are no specific problems with labour and delivery except occasional need for higher levels of opiate analgesia.
- Breastfeeding is allowed.
- Children of alcohol abusing parents are at risk of abuse and neglect and social services should be involved.

Q16. A woman attending a routine antenatal clinic inquires about epidural analgesia in labour. Unfortunately an anaesthetist cannot be found to answer her questions. Describe briefly how you would counsel the woman.

A16.

- Epidural analgesia is one of the most effective forms of pain relief in labour. It provides reliable and controlled analgesia which can be maintained or altered over time depending on the situation.
- The woman should be told that epidurals are usually sited when the woman is in the active phase of labour. A history of any back problems or injuries and of any spinal surgery should be taken to rule out any contraindications for the procedure. These include localized or generalized sepsis, coagulation disorders, severe hypovolaemia or congenital cardiac problems where hypotension may increase the right to left shunt.
- The epidural technique should be briefly explained to the woman including the fact that subcutaneous infiltration with a local anaesthetic is done prior to inserting the needle in the epidural space.
- The risks involved with epidural analgesia should be explained. This includes hypotension, which is treated with intravenous fluids and ephedrine if necessary.
- One in 150 women who have epidurals sited will suffer from headaches. This may range from mild self-limiting headaches to a postdural puncture headache, which is usually occipital and severe with photophobia and is worse on sitting or standing and relieved on lying flat. If it occurs, it usually requires strong analgesia in the form of opiates or may require a blood patch, which has an 80–90% success rate. There are usually no long-term sequelae of this complication.
- Neurological damage, which may be anything from a small numb patch to paraplegia may occur. This is usually temporary, lasting from a few days to weeks in 1 in 3000 women. In 1 in 10 000 women this may be permanent.
- The woman should be reassured that there is no evidence for backache being caused by epidural analgesia.
- There is an association of prolonged second stage of labour and an increased rate of instrumental deliveries with epidurals but no evidence of adverse neonatal effects.
- The woman should be warned that there is a risk of failure in which case alternative methods of analgesia would have to be tried.
- Explanatory leaflets should be given and, ideally, an appointment with an anaesthetist should be arranged.

Q17. A woman is referred to the antenatal clinic in her third pregnancy. Her previous obstetric history includes two preterm deliveries at 32 and 30 weeks, respectively. Critically appraise your management of her pregnancy.

A17.

- There is a substantial risk of recurrence of spontaneous preterm delivery, being 20% after one, and up to 35–40% with two previous preterm deliveries. It is thus important to manage the woman's next pregnancy carefully, ruling out the known causes of premature labour.
- An early first trimester dating scan is essential for accurate estimation of gestational age.
- Detailed screening for vaginal colonization with pathogenic organisms including group B *Streptococcus* and the presence of bacterial vaginosis should be done at the initial visit and then regularly throughout the pregnancy. The use of metronidazole in high risk women with bacterial vaginosis significantly lowers the risk of preterm birth by 60%. Similarly, testing for group B *Streptococcus* allows appropriate intrapartum prophylaxis.
- Asymptomatic bacteriuria causes an increased risk of preterm birth and should be treated with appropriate antibiotics.
- Transvaginal ultrasound to check for cervical length and signs of funneling should be undertaken to rule out cervical incompetence as a causative factor. The risk of preterm labour has been seen to increase by 4% when length is reduced to 11–20 mm. This risk increases to 15% at lengths of 10 mm. In cases of a short cervix, consideration should be given to the performance of a cervical cerclage procedure.
- No benefit has been proven with the use of oral tocolytics such as ritodrine.
- Cervicovaginal fibronectin testing may give an indication of preterm labour and may be used in centres where it is available.
- A thrombophilia screen may be indicated if there was evidence of placental dysfunction such as abruption, recurrent bleeding or intrauterine growth restriction in the previous pregnancies.
- It is important that the woman is kept under close surveillance at the hospital, with immediate admission in case of signs of recurrence of symptoms.

Screening Gp B, BV
Asymp. Bact
Cxl incomp.
Thrombophilia

Q18. A woman booking in her first pregnancy is found to have a platelet count of 100×10^9/L. This falls as the pregnancy advances until at 30 weeks it is down to 50×10^9/L. Justify your management.

A18.

- Thrombocytopaenia (TP) in pregnancy may be either gestational or autoimmune. It may also be due to acquired causes such as pre-eclampsia, or HELLP syndrome. Gestational thrombocytopaenia is a benign condition with a normal outcome for mother and baby. Autoimmune thrombocytopaenia is due to the destruction of platelets by autoantibodies directed against platelet surface antigens.
- It is difficult to distinguish between the two causes of thrombocytopaenia in pregnancy as antiplatelet antibodies (PAIgG) may be present in over 50% of women with gestational thrombocytopaenia.
- Autoimmune TP may be associated with fetal TP due to the passage of antibodies across the placenta. It may be associated with intracranial haemorrhage in 1–2% of cases.
- Serial monitoring of platelet count with a close liaison between the obstetrician, haematologist and neonatologist is essential.
- With a fall below 50×10^9, maternal treatment in the form of corticosteroids or intravenous immunoglobulins should be undertaken. 80% of patients respond to steroids within 3–6 weeks. The latter brings about a response in 4–6 days.
- The aim is to elevate the platelet count to above 50×10^9/L. Once the count has come up, the delivery should be expedited if term.
- In the rare event that the platelet counts fail to respond to these measures, a splenectomy should be considered.
- The overall incidence of TP in babies born to mothers with autoimmune TP is 11%, but the fetal risk of severe problems is extremely small. Because of this, vaginal delivery should be allowed unless there are obstetric indications for a caesarean section.
- All neonates should have their platelet counts assessed.
- There is a 1% risk of intracranial haemorrhage in fetuses with TP. In view of this, fetal blood samples and ventouse deliveries should be avoided.

Steroids, Ig, Splenectomy.

Q19. A routine full blood count in a pregnant woman taken at her booking visit reveals a haemoglobin of 7 g/dL, with the following red cell indices: MCV 96 fl, MCH 27 pg, MCHC 30 g/dL. Critically appraise your management.

MCV - 75-99

A19.

- The diagnosis in this case is megaloblastic anaemia. The two main causes of this are folate and vitamin B_{12} deficiencies, the former being the more frequent cause of anaemia than the latter.
- Diagnosis is confirmed by undertaking red cell folate levels and serum vitamin B_{12} levels. Other investigations that should be undertaken include Hb electrophoresis and a blood film examination.
- The importance of compliance with treatment should be stressed to the mother in view of the potential consequences of megaloblastic anaemia on the fetus. There is an association with periconceptual folic acid deficiency and neural tube defects, harelip and cleft palate. The neonate may also be affected with megaloblastic anaemia.
- Treatment should be started with 5 mg pteroylglutamic acid daily, and continued for several weeks after delivery. If there is no response, parenteral folic acid should be given. The importance of a dietary intake of fresh vegetables should be stressed as folate is rapidly destroyed by cooking. B_{12} is naturally found in all animal products and thus may be deficient in vegans.
- Women on antiepileptic medication and those with hereditary haemolytic conditions such as thalessaemia, sickle cell disease and spherocytosis are particularly vulnerable to folate deficiency and should be given a supplement of 5–10 mg folic acid daily.

Q20. A woman has a booking scan which reveals a monochorionic twin gestation. How will you plan the management of her pregnancy? A scan at 26 weeks reveals an increased amniotic fluid index in twin one and a decreased amniotic fluid index in twin two. How will you manage the rest of her pregnancy?

A20.

- Multiple gestations are associated with a sixfold increase in perinatal morbidity and mortality. Monochorionic twin pregnancies are particularly at risk of complications due to the presence of vascular connections between the fetoplacental circulation of each twin.
- There can be potentially handicapping complications of monochorionic twinning which include polyhydramnios and preterm delivery, and compromise or death of the donor twin in 'twin-to-twin transfusion syndromes' (TTTS). This includes severe oligohydramnios and intrauterine growth retardation and 'recipient' morbidity from cardiac dysfunction.
- These pregnancies should be scanned from 18 to 20 weeks gestation on a two weekly basis to try and avoid the most dismal prognosis of the most

Polyhydramnios
Preterm del
Oligohydramnios
IUGR TTTS

severe forms of TTTS. General advice should be given to these women regarding diet and iron and folic acid supplementation, and a close watch kept on the blood pressure.

- If on scan a monochorionic twin pregnancy shows polyhydramnios in one twin and oligohydramnios in the other, it is important to look for other signs of TTTS. These are markedly discordant growth with the larger twin (classically called the recipient) showing a large bladder on scan and features of congestive cardiac failure caused by hypervolaemia. These are in the form of hydrops, cardiomegaly and tricuspid regurgitation. The smaller 'donor' twin is often severely growth restricted, oliguric with oligohydramnios, giving rise to a 'stuck' appearance against the uterine wall. Doppler waveform changes also characteristically occur.
- On confirmation of the diagnosis of TTTS it is important to refer these women for further management to a fetal medicine referral centre used to dealing with these pregnancies. One of the options for management is aggressive serial amnio-reduction, with the repeated removal of large volumes of amniotic fluid (1–4 L) under ultrasound guidance. This reduces the risk of preterm labour secondary to polyhydramnios. A further therapeutic option is laser ablation of the vascular anastomosis using fetoscopy. Digoxin therapy may be used to improve cardiac function in the recipient twin. Most importantly, steroids should be administered if early delivery becomes imminent. It is important that the couple are fully counselled and informed about the prognosis. They should be put in touch with the multiple births foundation. ③Septostomy
  1. Serial amnio ④Selective feticide
     reduction
  2. Fetoscopic Laser ablation

Q21. You are a registrar on labour ward and are called to see a lady in labour. She is at term and is expecting twins with the first twin cephalic. She delivers the first twin uneventfully. Examination then reveals that the second twin is a transverse lie with intact membranes. How will you proceed with the rest of her labour?

A21.

- In the case of a second twin found to be a transverse lie after normal delivery of the first twin, it is important to assess the situation including any signs of fetal distress. In case of inadequate uterine activity, an oxytocin infusion should be started.
- As long as maternal and fetal condition is good, several options are available. Firstly, the lie can be corrected to a longitudinal lie. This can be done as an external cephalic version or an internal podalic version. External version gently turns the fetus so that it lies with the vertex above the pelvic brim. It is important to ensure good contractions in order for

the head to enter the pelvis before an amniotomy is undertaken, to avoid the risk of cord prolapse. Once an amniotomy is performed the baby is delivered by maternal effort. A scalp electrode will facilitate monitoring once the membranes are ruptured. The other option is to carry out an internal podalic version to breech presentation with intact membranes. It is done by locating a foot and then performing an amniotomy, followed by delivery of the baby by breech extraction.

- If the lie is not corrected by these manoeuvres, or in case of fetal distress, caesarean section should be performed. Epidural analgesia is associated with a higher success rate in case of version, the other advantage being ease of delivery if a caesarean section becomes necessary.
- After delivery of the second twin, active management of the third stage is essential because of the risk of postpartum haemorrhage. As a prophylaxis against uterine atony, an infusion of 10 iu syntocinon per hour should be started and continued for at least 4 h.

Q22. A routine mid-trimester scan on a woman reveals an anterior abdominal wall defect, in the form of an exomphalos. The couple are very worried and come to you for counselling and further management of the pregnancy. Justify your approach to this case.

A22.

- Exomphalos, or omphalocoele as it is also known, is a herniation of abdominal contents into a semitransparent sac through an abdominal defect. The umbilicus inserts into this sac rather than the anterior abdominal wall. The contents of the sac vary according to the size of the defect and its position on the anterior abdominal wall. These will contain bowel alone if it is a small defect and other organs like the liver, spleen and stomach if the defect is large. It occurs in around 1 in 2500 to 1 in 5000 pregnancies.
- Exomphalos can be associated with abnormal karyotype and abnormalities of other systems. Overall, 70% of exomphalos babies have associated congenital abnormalities, which include cardiac and neural tube defects. A detailed scan must be undertaken to look for these anomalies.
- In the presence of associated anomalies, the incidence of an abnormal fetal karyotype is 36%. In the absence of other anomalies this falls to 3%. It is thus important to counsel the parents to undergo fetal karyotyping. If multiple defects are present or in the presence of abnormal karyotype (mainly trisomy 18, 13 or 21), termination is offered to the parents.
- The prognosis is generally good in the presence of a normal karyotype with no associated abnormalities. The survival rate of normal infants is

in excess of 75%. Mortality occurs from prematurity, sepsis or short gut syndrome.

- Delivery should occur in a centre where neonatal medical and surgical expertise is on hand. Caesarean section does not confer any benefit and thus should not be undertaken unless there are obstetric indications.
- The object of immediate postdelivery care is to prevent heat and fluid loss and to prevent sepsis. The neonate is wrapped in a sterile bag containing warm electrolytes, plasma and antibiotics. Operative repair is undertaken as soon as the neonate's condition is stable. This can either be primary closure of small defects, or, where this is not possible due to the size of the defect, a silastic silo is used to cover the contents and sutured to the edge of the defect. This is gradually compressed over the next few days so that the contents of the sac are reduced.

Q23. Critically appraise the management of a pregnancy where a left-sided congenital diaphragmatic hernia has been diagnosed on ultra-sound scan at 16 weeks.

A23.

- Diaphragmatic hernias are a protrusion of the abdominal contents into the thoracic cavity. They occur in around 1 in 3500 live births. 80% of these are left sided and include the bowel, stomach and spleen. Right-sided hernias, which carry a worse prognosis, include the liver.
- Up to 50% of cases are associated with other anomalies, notably in the cardiovascular (ventricular septal defect, tetralogy of Fallot), gastrointest-inal, skeletal and genitourinary systems. It is thus important to look for other abnormalities.
- At least 10–20% are associated with aneuploidy, mainly trisomy 13, 18 and 21. Fetal karyotyping should therefore be recommended. Other syndromes associated with the condition are Pierre–Robin and Beckwith–Weidemann syndrome.
- Termination of pregnancy should be discussed with the parents, specially where aneuploidy or other structural anomalies are present.
- The main pathological effect of congenital diaphragmatic hernia is to prevent lung development. Polyhydramnios may occur due to impaired swallowing or obstruction of the upper gastrointestinal tract. There is evidence that the administration of steroids reduces severity of lung pathology and surfactant deficiency and should be administered prior to delivery.
- There is no benefit from open fetal surgery to repair the diaphragm or ligate the trachea.

- There is no indication for elective caesarean section. Induction may be considered in order to coincide delivery with the availability of neonatal support services. After delivery, treatment is centred on respiratory support until the lungs have stabilized sufficiently to tolerate surgical repair of the diaphragm. This may take up to 2 weeks. Extracorporeal membrane oxygenation (ECMO) is now being used to support respiration in these babies.
- The overall survival in isolated congenital diaphragmatic hernia is around 60%. Careful counselling by an experienced paediatrician familiar with the postnatal management of congenital diaphragmatic hernia is essential, as survival is still poor and postnatal management involves weeks of intensive care followed by long-term morbidity.
- It is important to reassure the parents that there is no increased recurrence risk except where the condition is part of a genetic syndrome.

Q24. A 26-year-old 16-week pregnant woman is found to have a fetal choroid plexus cyst on the booking scan. Justify your management, relevant to this finding.

A24.

- Choroid plexus cysts are small areas of cystic dilatation, seen in the choroid plexus of the lateral ventricles of the brain in 1–2% of fetuses. They usually disappear before the end of the second trimester.
- They may be associated with a risk of aneuploidy, mainly trisomy 18 (about 70% of cases of trisomy 18 have choroid plexus cysts). Other karyotypic abnormalities have also been reported.
- Because of this it is important to decide when to recommend a karyotyping procedure such as amniocentesis, with its inherent risk of miscarriage.
- The size of the cyst, whether unilateral or bilateral, or whether simple or complex does not alter the chance of chromosomal anomalies.
- It is important to consider personal and family history of chromosomal anomalies, and look for other anomalies on scan (major anomalies or soft markers).
- Mid-trimester serum screening should be advised.
- The most important factor here is maternal age. The risk of chromosomal anomalies associated with choroid plexus increases with increasing maternal age.
- The risk at an age of 31 years is about 1 in 280 (the usual cut-off risk at which karyotyping is recommended).

- At her age, with no other history or scan markers (at the initial scan as well as a 20–22 week detailed scan) the risk of chromosomal anomalies is too low to advise amniocentesis.
- The patient and her partner should be fully involved in the decision-making process.

Q25. A couple present to the antenatal clinic after a mid-trimester scan which has revealed ventriculomegaly. How will you counsel the couple and manage the pregnancy?

A25.

- Ventriculomegaly, also known as hydrocephalus, occurs when cerebro-spinal fluid collects intracranially, resulting in enlargement of the ventricular system.
- The first thing that should be ascertained is whether it is an isolated feature or if it is associated with other congenital anomalies. Isolated ventriculomegaly is associated in around 3% of cases with chromosomal anomalies. If associated with other defects, this figure rises to 36%. The most common associated anomaly (25–30%), is spina bifida, followed by other defects (central nervous system, renal, gastrointestinal) in 7–15% of cases. The couple should thus be counselled about karyotyping, and informed of the risks involved.
- The next thing to ascertain is the degree of ventriculomegaly, which may range from mild (> 10 mm cortical thickness + normal BPD) to severe (< 10 mm cortical thickness + abnormally increased BPD). If it is an isolated defect and is mild to moderate, serial scans will be needed to chart its progress. If the degree remained mild or if it disappeared altogether *in utero*, then the prognosis for neurodevelopment is excellent. However, if it progresses, the prognosis deteriorates.
- When associated with other defects or chromosomal abnormalities, the couple should be counselled about termination of the pregnancy by a senior obstetrician. In case they opt to continue the pregnancy, a decision has to be made, in conjunction with the parents, about mode of delivery. A poor prognosis may necessitate a decision against a caesarean delivery. In this case, cephalocentesis has to be considered to facilitate a vaginal delivery. This is invariably fatal for the fetus. If ventriculomegaly is isolated and has a good prognosis, it is better to decide on abdominal delivery.
- *In utero* surgery has not been shown to have a better outcome as compared to postnatal ventriculoperitoneal shunting. The parents will have to be warned about the need for surgery after delivery, with the attendant

risks of shunt infection, shunt obstruction and septicaemia. This is best done by a paediatric surgeon well versed with the procedure.

Q26. A woman is referred to you by her community midwife at 28 weeks gestation with a symphysiofundal height of 22 cm. Critically appraise your management.

A26.

- Symphysiofundal height estimation is a crude and often inaccurate method of detecting the small for gestational age (SGA) fetus. It is, however, a valuable method of detecting fetal growth restriction in the community. It is imperative to investigate such a case further and manage accordingly.

- A detailed ultrasound scan should be undertaken. Abdominal circumference and estimated fetal weight are measured to confirm the diagnosis of SGA. Customised ultrasound charts, taking into account maternal height, weight, ethnic group and parity should be used.

- Serial measurement for growth at an interval of 2 weeks should be undertaken to distinguish fetal growth restriction from constitutionally small babies. The latter will have normal growth velocity.

- If an SGA fetus is detected, a detailed scan to look for anomalies should be undertaken. Karyotyping should be offered to the couple, as often chromosomal abnormalities may be associated with this condition.

- Umbilical artery Doppler measurements and liquor volume are undertaken at regular intervals. In case of normal uterine artery Doppler's, fortnightly monitoring on an outpatient basis can be undertaken until fetal viability is reached.

- Steroids should be administered for lung maturity in case of the need for early delivery.

- Serial monitoring and conservative management under a fetal medicine expert should be undertaken as long as all the parameters are normal at least until 34 weeks.

- Delivery should be considered in case of reversed or absent end diastolic flow on uterine artery Dopplers at over 34 weeks gestation. If less than 34 weeks, admission and daily monitoring can continue as long as cardiotocographs, biophysical profiles and Dopplers are normal. If they become abnormal, delivery should be undertaken, usually by caesarean section.

- It is important to keep the woman and her partner informed of all decisions and the reasons for undertaking them.

Q27. A woman presents to delivery suite with premature contractions at 23 weeks gestation. A vaginal examination reveals her cervix to be 5 cm dilated with intact membranes. Critically appraise the steps you will take to manage the case.

A27.

- In this case, it is most likely that the patient will go on to deliver an extremely premature infant. It is important that all the issues of survival and prognosis at the margins of viability are discussed beforehand with the parents in order to prepare them for what may lie ahead.

- Every effort should be made to delay the birth, as chances of survival at this gestation improve by an average of 2% per day. Consideration should be given to transfer under tocolysis to a perinatal centre with facilities for neonatal intensive care.

- Steroids should be administered and tocolysis considered over the next 48 h in order for them to take effect. A full screen for chorioamnionitis should be undertaken with the administration of appropriate antibiotics if signs of infection are found.

- It is imperative that the parents should be counselled by a senior neonatologist as soon as possible. They should be made aware of the chances of survival if the baby were to be born, which differs from hospital to hospital. On average 50% survive at this gestation, of whom roughly 50% will be handicapped, half of them seriously. The chance of intact survival depends upon the presence or absence of a major intracranial lesion, severe lung disease or retinopathy of prematurity and the condition at delivery. On follow-up of these children, 20% will have special educational needs, with 25% functioning at a grade below expected and another 30% needing special classroom assistance.

- The parents should be counselled about the decision to undertake active resuscitation of the baby. Their wishes should be taken into account, though they must be made aware that the plan may have to be changed depending upon circumstances. Resuscitation of apnoeic, floppy and non-responsive babies may have to be abandoned, whereas, even if a decision has been made beforehand not to actively resuscitate, it may have to be changed in case of a vigorous, responsive baby.

- It is important that a senior neonatologist is present at delivery. The parents should be informed of events at each step.

- The issue of management of babies at the margins of viability is still controversial and is changing day to day. It is however, imperative to undertake all decisions and measures with the parents' informed consent.

Q28. A woman books at 9 weeks in her second pregnancy, having had a caesarean section in her previous pregnancy. Critically appraise how you will decide on the mode of delivery.

A28.

- In the case of a woman with a previous caesarean section scar, mode of delivery in the next pregnancy should be decided after going over all the circumstances of the first delivery and should be an informed choice by the woman.
- It is important to review the case notes of the previous delivery, and to obtain them if the delivery was conducted elsewhere. This is mainly to differentiate between classical and lower transverse scars, because the former is associated with a much higher risk of uterine rupture before the onset of labour. In the rare case of a classical uterine scar it is advisable to undergo an elective caesarean delivery at 38 weeks.
- The woman should be counselled about the success rates of vaginal birth after caesarean (VBAC), which is approximately 75% for all patients with a prior caesarean section scar, ranging from 67% for patients with prior failure to progress in labour to 85% for patients with a non-recurring indication such as breech presentation.
- The advantages of VBAC are a shorter hospital stay with less morbidity, which includes lower incidences of postpartum transfusions and febrile episodes as compared to even an elective caesarean section.
- On the other hand, there is a higher morbidity associated with emergency caesarean sections after failed trial of vaginal birth as compared to elective caesarean sections, and the woman should be made aware of this.
- Uterine rupture occurs in approximately 1 : 100 cases of trial of scar.
- In accordance with current policies of risk management, the woman should be asked to sign a consent form for whatever mode of delivery she decides upon, to signify that she has made an informed choice.
- Whatever route of delivery is chosen, a history of previous caesarean section elevates the risk to both mother and baby. Febrile and thromboembolic complications, uterine rupture and hysterectomy are all more common in women with a history of previous caesarean section, regardless of mode of delivery in the subsequent pregnancy.

Q29. Evaluate how you could reduce the morbidity and mortality associated with caesarean sections.

A29.

- There is a four-to fivefold increase in maternal mortality at caesarean section as compared to vaginal deliveries, the main causes being pulmonary embolism, hypertension, haemorrhage, sepsis and anaesthetic complications. With proper planning and senior obstetric input, this can be considerably reduced.
- Proper planning is essential, with a complete knowledge of the previous obstetric, medical and surgical history, and that of any previous anaesthetic complications, allergies, previous postpartum haemorrhage, position of fetus and placental site.
- All women undergoing caesarean section should have a risk assessment for thrombosis and the type of thromboprophylaxis used should be based on this, in accordance with RCOG guidelines.
- The risk of haemorrhage is increased in cases of placenta praevia, previous history of postpartum haemorrhage, obesity, prolonged second stage of labour, pre-eclampsia, general anaesthesia, amnionitis, preterm caesarean and classical uterine incisions. The placental site should be checked by ultrasound scan in women undergoing repeat caesarean sections. An anterior placenta praevia with a previous caesarean scar increases the risk of placenta accreta, and thus the patient should be forewarned, with consent for a caesarean hysterectomy provisionally obtained before the operation. It is mandatory that a senior obstetrician be present and adequate amount of blood cross-matched.
- Correct surgical technique will prevent a lot of morbidity in the form of haemorrhage and visceral damage. Wide lateral dissection of the bladder should be avoided. The uterine incision should be cut concave upwards, rather than by tearing the uterus digitally. Spontaneous expulsion of the placenta reduces fetomaternal haemorrhage. Oxytocic drugs should be used to reduce blood loss in the third stage.
- Infection is a major cause of morbidity in both elective and emergency caesarean sections. Predisposing factors are prolonged rupture of membranes, maternal obesity, and isolation of organisms from the upper vaginal tract such as β-haemolytic *Streptococcus* and bacterial vaginosis. Antibiotic prophylaxis causes a significant reduction in postoperative infectious morbidity.

Q30. Critically appraise the surgical techniques, which may improve the outcome of caesarean sections.

A30.

- Good surgical technique is a key factor in reducing the morbidity and mortality associated with caesarean sections.
- The skin incision should ideally be made in the pelvic groove, 2 cm above the pubic symphysis. Sharp facial dissection is advisable for repeat caesarean sections, with the parietal peritoneum being opened high anteriorly to avoid excising an unexpectedly high bladder.
- In obstructed second stage of labour, the low transverse uterine incision should be made high to avoid opening into the vagina. Wide lateral dissection of the bladder should be avoided, and the uterine incision should be cut concave upwards rather than by tearing digitally.
- The fetal head should be delivered through the uterine incision in the occipitoanterior position, disengaging it from the pelvis and rotating it prior to delivery, if in a posterior or transverse position.
- Spontaneous expulsion of the placenta should be allowed rather than shearing it manually, thus increasing the risk of haemorrhage and subsequent infection.
- Oxytocic agents should be used in the third stage of labour, preferably intravenous oxytocin. In case of uterine atony, vigorous massage of the uterus along with intramyometrial injections of carboprost (prostaglandin $F_{2\alpha}$), direct pressure over the bleeding placental surface and the use of figure-of-eight sutures in the placental bed should be used. Senior help should be summoned in case of persistent haemorrhage and consideration of bilateral ligation of the uterine arteries or a B-Lynch brace suture used to stem the haemorrhage.

Q31. You are the registrar on call for labour ward and are called to see a patient in labour by her midwife. She is primiparous at term, and has progressed from 7 cm to 10 cm cervical dilatation in 5 h. She has been pushing for an hour and a half without success. Critically appraise your management.

A31.

- When called upon to deal with a case of dystocia in labour, it is important to take into account various factors before deciding on the mode of delivery.
- The antenatal history should be quickly ascertained from the notes, and any recent ultrasound scans reviewed which may indicate a cause for the dystocia such as macrosomia.

- The fetal cardiotocograph should be checked to make sure there are no signs of fetal distress.
- A complete abdominal and vaginal examination is then done to palpate duration, frequency and strength of uterine contractions, and to see if any fifths of the head can be palpated per abdomen. A vaginal examination to confirm full dilatation and to ascertain station of the vertex as well as its position and any asynclitism is undertaken. All the findings should be clearly documented and signed.
- If it is felt that inadequate uterine activity is a contributing factor in the delay of the second stage, an oxytocin drip should be started if a vaginal delivery is felt to be feasible. The decision to undertake an instrumental delivery will depend on the results of the abdominal and vaginal examinations. If the head is deeply engaged and not palpable on an abdominal examination, an instrumental delivery should be attempted. In view of the 'secondary arrest' pattern of labour, it may be prudent to conduct this in the operating theatre, with staff on standby for a caesarean section in case of failure of instrumental delivery. Adequate analgesia in the form of epidural, spinal or pudendal block should be ensured.
- In case of more than a fifth of the head being palpable abdominally, a caesarean section should be carried out. All decisions should be discussed thoroughly with the patient and her partner and informed consent taken.

Q32. A woman in her first pregnancy is seen in the antenatal clinic at 41 weeks, having had no previous problems in the pregnancy. Outline your plan of management and justify the steps you would take.
A32.

- Around 10% of all pregnant women will undergo a prolonged pregnancy, which is 42 completed weeks of gestation or more. It is important to be aware of the risks involved with prolonged pregnancies and how to manage them.
- The correct gestation should be checked. This is greatly facilitated if an early scan has been carried out in the pregnancy to confirm dates.
- Induction of labour should be done at 41+ weeks. This is supported by randomized controlled trials which have shown a reduction in perinatal mortality, decreased meconium staining of the amniotic fluid, and a reduction in the caesarean section rate compared to conservative management.
- The woman and her partner should be counselled about the reasons for induction and their wishes should be taken into consideration.

- Intrapartum fetal death is four times more common and early neonatal death three times as common in infants born after 42 weeks. The rate of neonatal seizures in infants born after 41 weeks is also more common.
- Infants born beyond 41 weeks of gestation show a higher rate of sudden infant death syndrome.
- A complete assessment should be undertaken in the antenatal clinic, which ought to include a clinical estimation of growth, presentation and a vaginal assessment to give a Bishop's score. The mode of induction should preferably be with prostaglandins.
- Around 30% of women with a prolonged pregnancy will opt for conservative management. In this case, close fetal surveillance should be carried out. This may include biophysical scoring or simpler methods such as measuring the amniotic fluid index along with cardiotocography.
- Successful management of these pregnancies depends upon effective counselling of the women and their full participation in the decision-making process.

Q33. Clinical risk management is becoming more and more important in the practice of obstetrics. Justify this statement and explain how you would ensure risk management in your unit.

A33.

- Clinical risk management is defined as the identification, analysis and control of risks in order to prevent adverse events from occurring and to ensure quality of care for the patient. As patient awareness and expectations from the health service rises this plays more and more of a central role in ensuring patient satisfaction and optimum care.
- It is important to have outlined within an obstetric unit, clinical guidelines, which should be followed and regularly updated. They should undergo regular audit to see that they are adhered to.
- Clinical incident reporting in the atmosphere of a 'no blame culture' is important in identifying adverse events and to analyse the reasons for such an occurrence. This ensures that guidelines are put into place to prevent such an occurrence in future.
- Adequate means of communication between junior and senior medical and midwifery staff should be in place so that potential problems can be prevented. It is important that senior medical staff are informed of any high risk patients and are involved in their care to ensure the best possible outcome. This includes recognizing the importance of dedicated consultant sessions on labour ward.

- Audit, education and professional assessments of medical and midwifery staff to ensure competence in the management of patients and the performance of surgical skills is important.
- Good record keeping is mandatory and should be an essential prerequisite of all obstetric units. All entries should be accurately timed, dated and signed with the signatory clearly identifiable.
- It is important to have skilled and fully trained staff with an appropriate midwife to patient ratio.
- 'Practice drills' which is the practice of rehearsing a response to particular emergencies such as shoulder dystocia or obstetric haemorrhage has been shown to improve performance when such emergencies arise in real life. They should be made a part of routine labour ward management.

Q34. A couple with a 2-year-old child with cerebral palsy come to you to find out if the management of the labour could have been responsible for the condition. They vaguely recollect an abnormal cardiotocograph in labour, which led to an emergency caesarean section. Their child was on the neonatal intensive care unit for a few weeks. Critically appraise the steps you will take to counsel the couple.

A34.

- The issue of cerebral palsy which may be secondary to intrapartum events is an extremely sensitive one. It needs to be handled carefully, by a senior obstetrician, preferably in the presence of a senior neonatologist familiar with the case.
- First and foremost, the case records should be carefully perused before meeting the couple. This includes the antenatal history, intrapartum events and the neonatal course, noting any interventions taken.
- One should ascertain the gestation at which the child was delivered, including any history of antenatal problems such as intrauterine growth restriction, major and multiple congenital or metabolic abnormalities, or the presence of microcephaly at birth. The latter should point to causes other than acute intrapartum hypoxia.
- The nature of any intrapartum problems along with interventions should be noted. The results of any fetal blood samples or cord blood arterial pH and base deficit are important and point towards a profound metabolic or mixed acidaemia if the umbilical artery pH <7.00 or base deficit >12 mmol/L.
- Signs of hypoxic ischaemic encephalopathy in the neonatal period include marked hypotonia, seizures, coma and the requirement of artificial ventilation. Moderate to severe encephalopathy (grade II–III) confer an in-

Major
1. Cord blood pH <7, BE ≥ 12 mmol
2. Early onset severe/mod NE in ≥ 34 wks
3. Spastic / dyskinetic

creased risk of serious handicap. It should be borne in mind however, that it is very uncommon to have moderate to severe encephalopathy following a non-reassuring cardiotocograph, and conversely, many cases of severe neonatal encephalopathy are not associated with intrapartum hypoxaemia.

- Spastic quadriplegia and dyskinetic cerebral palsy are the only subtypes of cerebral palsy associated with acute hypoxic intrapartum events. Hemiplegic cerebral palsy, spastic diplegia and ataxia are not associated with acute intrapartum events.
- The presence of neonatal cranial ultrasound, MRI or EEGs to predict signs of acute hypoxaemia should be looked for. Cerebral oedema on cranial ultrasound appears as an increase in echodensity, loss of anatomical landmarks and compression of the ventricles along with periventricular haemorrhage. MRI may diagnose cerebral arterial infarcts, cortical atrophy and basal ganglion lesions.
- Any risk factors for an antenatal cause of cerebral palsy should be assessed. These include early imaging evidence of long-standing neurological abnormalities such as ventriculomegaly or porencephaly.
- Other questions that need to be answered are whether there was a sentinel hypoxic event and would quicker delivery of the baby have prevented or ameliorated the outcome.
- Once all the facts of the case have been ascertained, the parents should be informed of them in a sympathetic manner. In case they wish to pursue the matter further or lodge a complaint, they should be put in touch with the appropriate authorities.

Q35. A woman complains of severe dyspareunia at a routine 6-week postnatal appointment following a normal vaginal delivery. Justify your investigations and management.

A35.

- Persisting dyspareunia can be a source of considerable postnatal morbidity and leads not only to physical discomfort but occasionally to psychological problems in the form of depression. The complaint should be thoroughly investigated and treated in a sympathetic manner.
- A detailed history of the mode of delivery and the onset of symptoms should be taken. This should include the presence of any perineal tear or episiotomy and how this was sutured. The case notes should be reviewed. The specific type of symptom should be ascertained, including the presence of superficial or deep dyspareunia, and if it is associated with vaginal bleeding, discharge or pelvic pain.

minor —   1. Bentinel hypoxic event
2. Sudden deliv of CTG
3. APGAR 0-6 > 5 min
4. multi System ab—

Scar
lufn.
Lubrication

- A thorough examination, both general and local, is then undertaken, with inspection of the vulva, vagina and perineum, looking for signs of tenderness, granulation tissue or breakdown of a previous repair. In case of signs of infection, a culture swab should be taken, including high and low vaginal and endocervical swabs. A gentle bimanual pelvic examination is done, looking for signs of tenderness and any pelvic masses. A per-rectal examination will complete the evaluation.
- If perineal scarring, breakdown of a repair or granulation tissue is the cause of the pain, an examination under anaesthesia and refashioning of the repair is done, excising any scar tissue present. A course of antibiotics should be given prior to the procedure in case of overt infection.
- A Fenton's procedure may be necessary in certain cases.
- In case of deep dyspareunia, a diagnostic laparoscopy may be considered, taking care to treat any pelvic infections beforehand.
- Vaginal dryness may be a cause of dyspareunia, especially in case of lactating mothers. Lubrication prior to intercourse should be advocated to the couple.

Q36. A woman in her second pregnancy comes to you wanting to know about the potential risks and benefits of collecting cord blood for banking of haemopoietic stem cells (HSC) at the time of delivery. She has a healthy 3-year-old child and there is no history of any genetic or acquired diseases in the family. How will you counsel her?
A36.

- Cord blood represents a rich source of haemopoietic stem cells which can potentially be used in HLA compatible recipients in case of relapsed lymphoblastic leukaemia in children. It may also be a source of other stem cells, which may in the future benefit other conditions such as degenerative diseases like Alzheimer's disease, or genetic diseases such as cystic fibrosis or muscular dystrophy. However, at the present time, such therapies are not proven.
- One should inform the patient that cord blood is a good source of HSC, but not of other stem cells.
- It is possible to make altruistic donations for cord blood banking, but this is confined to certain centres in the country.
- Cord blood collection and storage is recommended for siblings born into a family where there is a known genetic disease amenable to HSC transplantation.
- However, in the absence of any known conditions in the family or in siblings which may benefit from HSC transplantation, it is highly unlikely

that stored cord blood will be needed. In view of the logistic problems of collection, this is not done routinely on the NHS, though some commercial companies are undertaking this venture at a cost.

- Cord blood needs to be collected in the third stage of labour with the placenta still attached *in utero*. This will distract the midwife or obstetrician from dealing appropriately with the labour, with all the inherent potential risks. It is thus not advisable on a routine basis.
- Cord blood banking has recently gained a lot of media attention. It is not recommended unless there is a particular indication as most of the potential benefits are still only theoretical.

Q37. Discuss the specific factors to be taken into consideration when planning an elective caesarean section at 39 weeks in a patient with an anterior placenta praevia, who has had two previous caesarean sections.
A37.

- The combination of anterior placenta praevia and previous caesarean section scars increases the possibility of morbidly adherent placenta.
- There are factors specific to the:

Patient:

- Counselling about the risk of severe haemorrhage ⊥ the need for hysterectomy.
- This should be discussed antenatally (not immediately preoperative) and documented.

Obstetrician:

- Should be experienced (consultant level).
- Good assistant should be available.

Anaesthetist:

- Should be experienced (consultant level).
- GA is to be recommended in view of the high risk of major bleeding.

Blood bank:

- At least 4 units of blood should be cross-matched and ready in theatre.
- Blood bank should be informed about the proposed time of procedure and the high chance of needing more blood/clotting factors.

Q38. Critically discuss the value of urine testing in pregnancy.
A38.

- Urine testing in pregnancy as a routine test and as a test indicated in specific circumstances.

Routine urine culture at the booking visit:
- To identify asymptomatic bacteriuria (ASB) (>100 000 organisms/mL).
- ASB is associated with a 30% chance of developing symptomatic UTI (pyelonephritis) later in pregnancy (vs. 0.2–2% in women with no ASB).
- Pyelonephritis in pregnancy can be serious, even fatal, and may lead to septic shock ARDS, and preterm labour.
- A week's course of antibiotics will sterilize urine in 65–90% of patients with ASB and prevent 80% of cases of pyelonephritis.

Routine urine testing for glucose:
- Is an inefficient screening test of gestational diabetes (sensitivity 27%, positive predictive value 7%).
- Should indicate a GTT only if at least 3+.

Routine urine testing for protein:
- May indicate cystitis, but often false positive.
- If heavy and persistent proteinuria may indicate renal pathology.
- May be associated with high BP (PET).

Indicated urine testing:
- Quantitative proteinuria in case of pregnancy-induced hypertension.
- Culture in case of symptoms of UTI.
- VMA in cases of suspected phaeochromocytoma.
- As a rapid toxicology screen in cases of suspected drug abuse.

Q39. Critically discuss the drugs used for thromboprophylaxis in obstetric practice.

A39.
- The risk of thromboembolism (TE) is increased in pregnancy, due to the physiological prothrombotic changes. This risk is particularly increased in women who have an inherent increased risk.

Warfarin:
- Warfarin crosses the placenta, is teratogenic and must therefore be avoided during the first trimester.
- The period of risk is *between the sixth and twelfth week* of gestation, so conception on warfarin therapy is not dangerous, provided the warfarin is replaced by heparin within 2 weeks of the first missed period.
- There is a significant risk of both maternal (retroplacental) and fetal (intracerebral) bleeding when used in the *third trimester*, and particularly after 36 weeks.
- The only indication for warfarin use in pregnancy is for thromboprophylaxis in women with metal prosthetic heart valve replacements. These women require full anticoagulation throughout pregnancy.

Heparin:
- This is available as unfractionated (UH) or low molecular weight (LMWH).
- Does not cross the placenta.
- The associated incidence of symptomatic osteoporosis may be as high as 2%. However, bone density improves once heparin therapy is discontinued.
- Thrombocytopaenia is another rare but potentially dangerous side-effect.
- LMWH has higher bioavailability than UH and needs once only administration. It also possibly has fewer side-effects (bleeding and thrombocytopaenia).

Aspirin
- Antiplatelet therapy has been shown to be effective in reducing the risk of venous thrombosis in surgical and medical patients.
- The use of aspirin as thromboprophylaxis in pregnancy has never been submitted to randomized controlled trial but it is known that low-dose aspirin is safe in pregnancy.
- It does not seem unreasonable therefore to use aspirin in situations where the risk of thrombosis is not deemed high enough to warrant subcutaneous heparin.
- Pharmacological thromboprophylaxis is not without risk. It should be used only when, after assessment of individual risk, it is thought that the perceived benefits (prevention of TE) outweigh the risks.

Q40. A pregnant woman at 10 weeks gestation had been in contact with a child who developed chickenpox 2 days later. Justify your advice and management.

A40.
- The infectivity period starts 2 days before appearance of the rash (until the vesicles are dry). Therefore, the child was infective when he came in contact with the patient.
- Enquiry should be made from her about past history of chickenpox. If there is definite history then she is immune and can be reassured. If there is no history or she is uncertain, then she should have blood taken and tested for varicella antibodies (IgG).
- Until her varicella status is sorted out, the patient should be advised not to come in contact with pregnant women, in case she is infective. Thus she should not come to the antenatal clinic during that time.
- If she is found not to be immune, she should to be given varicella-zoster immunoglobulins (VZIG) as soon as practically possible. VZIG will either

prevent or attenuate maternal/fetal varicella infection if given up to 10 days after exposure.

- Detection of VZ IgM in maternal serum indicates primary VZ infection. When occurring in the first 20 weeks of pregnancy, primary infection carries a 2% risk of congenital varicella infection (includes skin scarring, eye defects, hyperplasia of limbs, neurological abnormalities). Referral to a specialist centre for detailed ultrasound scan at 16 weeks gestation or 5 weeks after infection, whichever is sooner, should be considered.
- Neonatal ophthalmic examination should be organized at birth.
- Maternal varicella infection carries the risk of maternal varicella pneumonia, which complicates up to 10% of cases and has a mortality rate of up to 1%. Therefore, if she is not immune, she should be advised to report any rash or chest symptoms to her doctor, even if she had received VZIG.

Chapter 2
Medical disorders in pregnancy

Chapter 2: Questions

Answers are on pp. 58–76

Q41. A woman comes to your prepregnancy clinic seeking advice. She is 20 years old and suffers from cystic fibrosis. Critically appraise your management.

Q42. Describe the preconceptual counselling that you would offer a 25-year-old nulliparous woman whose natural father suffers from haemophilia A (factor VIII deficiency).

Q43. A 26-year-old woman comes to the prepregnancy assessment clinic. She suffers from epilepsy and is trying to conceive for the first time. What particular advice would you offer her?

Q44. A 38-year-old insulin-dependent diabetic presents to you for advice. She wants to attempt a first pregnancy. She is a poorly controlled diabetic. What advice would you give her?

Q45. A woman books in the first trimester of her pregnancy. She has a history of heart disease. How will you manage her pregnancy?

Q46. Critically discuss the management of thyrotoxicosis in pregnancy.

Q47. A 35-year-old woman at 26 weeks gestation presents with signs and symptoms consistent with pulmonary embolism. Critically appraise your management.

Q48. A woman attending for a routine antenatal appointment complains of generalized itching. There is no sign of a rash or allergy and she is not on any medication. She is found to have mild jaundice and is 32 weeks into her pregnancy. Critically appraise your investigations and management.

Q49. A woman books in her first pregnancy at 6 weeks gestation. She suffers from sickle cell disease and wants to know the consequences of this on her pregnancy and on the fetus. She is married to her first cousin. Justify the counselling you would give her, and your management of her pregnancy.

Q50. You are asked to see a woman on the postnatal ward, who has delivered a baby by caesarean section 3 days ago and seems to be severely depressed. Critically appraise how you will manage this situation?

Q51. A woman whose first child suffers from β-thalassaemia is now 8 weeks into her second pregnancy. She is very worried about the baby and comes to you for advice. No one else is affected in her immediate family. Justify the advice and counselling you will impart to her.

Q52. A 32-year-old woman at 20 weeks into her first pregnancy undergoes colposcopic examination for postcoital bleeding. She is found to have a growth on her cervix, which is later clinically staged to be a IIIb squamous cell carcinoma. Critically appraise your subsequent management.

Q53. A 28-year-old woman who has been treated for breast cancer a year ago, comes to you for advice. She does not have any children and is very keen on starting a family. She has had adjuvant chemotherapy and is currently on tamoxifen. Critically appraise the advice you will impart to her.

Q54. A 27-year-old woman has recently undergone a renal transplantation and is contemplating a pregnancy. What advice, specific to her condition, would you give her?

Q55. A 36-year-old woman who is pregnant for the first time is a severe asthmatic. What particular precautions will you take while managing her pregnancy?

Q56. 'Low molecular weight heparins are better than conventional heparin in the prevention and treatment of thromboembolic episodes'. Justify this statement.

Q57. A patient is referred to you at 26 weeks gestation. She has recently come to the UK from abroad and has been diagnosed to be suffering from pulmonary tuberculosis. Evaluate your management plan.

Q58. Critically appraise the use of anticoagulants in pregnant women with prosthetic heart valves.

Q59. One week after a normal delivery, a previously healthy woman starts complaining of breathlessness and chest pain. She has an echocardiogram, suggesting the diagnosis of cardiomyopathy. Outline the principles of management.

Q60. A woman suffering from systemic lupus nephritis wishes to start a family. Critically appraise the advice you will give her and your proposed management of her pregnancy.

Chapter 2: **Answers**

Q41. A woman comes to your prepregnancy clinic seeking advice. She is 20 years old and suffers from cystic fibrosis. Critically appraise your management.

A41.

- Cystic fibrosis is the commonest inherited genetic condition in white Caucasians. The mutated gene is carried on chromosome 7 and is carried by around 1 in 25 of the population. The incidence per live birth is 1 in 2500.

- The mutated gene results in defective production of a large protein located on the membrane of apical epithelial cells. Thick secretions are produced in the exocrine glands which cause organ damage.

- It is important in this case to fully discuss the effect of a pregnancy on the woman's health, the chances of a successful pregnancy outcome and the chance of inheritance of the condition. As cystic fibrosis is inherited in an autosomal recessive pattern, all offspring are obligate carriers but will not be affected unless the male partner carries the mutated gene for the condition. If the father is a carrier then the offspring will have a 1 in 2 chance of being affected. Paternal screening is thus essential before any questions regarding inheritance can be answered.

- Pregnancy is well tolerated if prepregnancy health is good. The best predictor of a favourable outcome for mother and baby is forced expiratory volume in 1 min (FEV_1). Women with severe disease, i.e. FEV_1 <60%, should be counselled about the significant mortality rate, which is 12% over the first 6 months after delivery. Women should be advised to achieve a body weight within 15% of the ideal.

- Modification of drug therapy may be required under the supervision of the respiratory physicians. Aminoglycosides are associated with fetal renal ototoxicity and quinolones have an antagonistic effect on folate metabolism. In women with pancreatic insufficiency resulting in diabetes, the achievement of tight diabetic control is essential to minimize the risk of congenital abnormalities.

- The male partner carrier status should be determined. If he is found to be a carrier, the options are either IVF and preimplantation genetic diagnosis or antenatal diagnosis to determine whether the fetus is affected or not. The couple should be thoroughly counselled and informed about the perinatal death rate of 11.5%, the main contributing factor being prematurity and preterm delivery.

Q42. Describe the preconceptual counselling that you would offer a 25-year-old nulliparous woman whose natural father suffers from haemophilia A (factor VIII deficiency).

A42.

- Haemophilia A is the most commonly inherited severe bleeding disorder. It is a sex-linked disorder, with the woman most likely being an obligate carrier. Carriers of haemophilia usually have factor VIII levels around 50%.
- All women who are carriers of haemophilia should undergo prepregnancy counselling including genetic counselling. They have a 50% chance of giving birth to a haemophilic child if it is male or a carrier if it is female.
- Severely affected males have spontaneous bleeds into muscles or joints, those mildly affected may only bleed after major surgery or trauma. If the woman was to go ahead with the pregnancy she should be offered prenatal diagnosis in the form of chorionic villus biopsy at 11–14 weeks. However, even this procedure carries a risk of bleeding. Alternatively, amniocentesis or fetal blood sampling may be used.
- Ultrasound scans can distinguish fetal sex. Gender preselection is possible through IVF and preimplantation genetic diagnosis.
- Prepregnancy planning should include vaccination against hepatitis A and B. Pregnancies should be managed in hospitals where there is a haemophilia centre with a close liaison between the obstetrician and haemophilia team.
- If maternal factor VIII remains low at 36 weeks then treatment with recombinant factor VIII may be considered.
- Epidural anaesthesia may be used if coagulation factors have been corrected. There is an increased risk of postpartum haemorrhage and in this case desmopressin can be used.
- If the fetus is male or a known haemophiliac traumatic vaginal delivery should be avoided. Ventouse delivery is contraindicated and maternal perineal trauma is avoided. In the infant, intramuscular injections are avoided and cord blood taken for a clotting factor assay.
- The couple should be put in touch with support groups consisting of parents bringing up children with the condition. As haemophilia care improves, most couples are now willing to contemplate bringing up a child with haemophilia.

Q43. A 26-year-old woman comes to the prepregnancy assessment clinic. She suffers from epilepsy and is trying to conceive for the first time. What particular advice would you offer her?

A43.

- It is important to go into a detailed history including duration, type and severity of epilepsy and current medication.
- All anticonvulsant drugs cross the placenta and can be teratogenic. These include phenytoin, carbamazepine, sodium valproate, primidone and phenobarbitone. The major malformations are neural tube defects, particularly with valproate (1–2%) and carbamazepine (0.5%–1%); orofacial clefts (phenytoin); and congenital heart defects (phenytoin and valproate). Minor malformations include dysmorphic features, hypertelorism and nail hypoplasia.
- The risk increases if more than one drug is used. The risk for one drug is 6–7%, for two drugs simultaneously used is 15% and for a combination of three drugs can be as high as 50%. Thus, if at all possible prepregnancy control should be sought with one drug. Control should be optimized prior to pregnancy.
- She should take preconceptual folic acid in a dose of 5 mg daily at least 12 weeks prior to conception. This should be continued throughout the pregnancy as there is a risk of folate deficiency anaemia even when the risk of neural tube defects occurring is past.
- The child has a higher risk of developing epilepsy, which is 4% if either parent has epilepsy, and 15–20% if both parents are sufferers.
- Women who are fit free for many years may wish to discontinue their medication preconceptually and in the first trimester. This should be a fully informed decision and should be jointly undertaken with the attending physician.

Q44. A 38-year-old insulin-dependent diabetic presents to you for advice. She wants to attempt a first pregnancy. She is a poorly controlled diabetic. What advice would you give her?

A44.

- In a case of an insulin-dependant diabetic desiring to become pregnant, it is imperative to give accurate prepregnancy advice so that optimal control can be achieved, and when the woman does become pregnant, adequate monitoring of the pregnancy can be undertaken.

- All the complications of diabetes in pregnancy are increased manifold if adequate glycaemic control is not achieved. Thus it is important to liaise with the endocrinologist so that near normoglycaemia is achieved.
- Prepregnancy counselling gives an opportunity for optimal diabetic control prior to pregnancy and assessment of the presence and severity of complications.
- There is an increased risk of congenital malformations in the fetus and the risk is associated with the HbA_{1c} levels around the time of conception. Women with $HbA_{1c} < 8\%$ have a risk of 5%, but in those with levels of $>10\%$, the risk is as high as 25%. Abnormalities include congenital heart defects, skeletal and neural tube defects and sacral agenesis.
- The requirements of insulin increase as pregnancy advances. Women with diabetic nephropathy and retinopathy may experience a worsening of their symptoms. Oral hypoglycaemic drugs should be avoided in pregnancy as they cross the placenta.
- The woman should be warned of the higher risk of complications such as pre-eclampsia, macrosomia and shoulder dystocia at delivery.
- Regular ultrasound scans to detect macrosomia and polyhydramnios are usually advised. Well-controlled diabetics are now allowed to go to term in the hope of spontaneous onset of labour.
- Pregnancy in women with pre-existing diabetes mellitus is associated with high risks and requires careful liaison between obstetricians, endocrinologists, nurses, dietitians and midwives, with the cooperation of the patient involved.

Q45. A woman books in the first trimester of her pregnancy. She has a history of heart disease. How will you manage her pregnancy?
A45.
- Cardiac disease is an important cause of maternal mortality in the UK. Widespread haemodynamic changes occur in pregnancy which are normally well tolerated. However, in those with cardiac disease these adaptations can place the woman at considerable risk of morbidity and mortality.
- In order to successfully manage the pregnant woman with heart disease, a team approach is required involving the obstetrician, cardiologist, anaesthetist, physician and cardiothoracic surgeon.
- It is important to go into details into the woman's past history including type of cardiac problem, any corrective surgery or presence of heart valves if relevant, and any medication being taken.

- Regurgitant valvular disease such as mitral or aortic regurgitation is usually well tolerated in pregnancy because the fall in peripheral resistance improves forward flow and lessens regurgitation. However, the stenotic lesions worsen in pregnancy.
- Patients with pulmonary hypertension, whether primary or secondary, are at particular risk because of a precarious balance between their systemic and pulmonary vascular resistance. In Eisenmenger's syndrome, pregnancy becomes risky with high fetal and maternal mortality rates. Maternal deaths usually occur during labour or in the postpartum period. Such women should be strongly advised against pregnancy or offered a termination. The risk of maternal mortality in case of a termination is 7% as compared to 50% in case of continuing with the pregnancy.
- During pregnancy factors which may cause cardiac decompensation should be avoided, e.g. anaemia, infections, dysarrythmias and hypertension.
- Serial ultrasound scans to monitor fetal growth are important in women with severe cardiac disease and cyanotic congenital heart disease. A detailed mid-trimester scan along with an echocardiogram should be performed to rule out any congenital heart disease in the fetus.
- A vaginal delivery with effective analgesia and a short second stage is usually preferred with the reservation of caesarean sections for obstetric indications or specific cardiac conditions. Blood loss during delivery should be minimized.
- The choice of anaesthesia depends upon maternal cardiac status. With adequate circulatory reserve, epidural anaesthesia is well tolerated. It should be used with extreme caution in patients with restricted cardiac output or right to left shunts. In these, general anaesthesia is the safer option.
- Antibiotic prophylaxis should be given to women at high risk for endocarditis.
- Thromboembolic complications increase in patients with prosthetic heart valves and they should be anticoagulated for the whole of the pregnancy.

Q46. Critically discuss the management of thyrotoxicosis in pregnancy.
A46.
- Thyrotoxicosis complicates 1:500 pregnancies with 50% of women having a positive family history of autoimmune disease. Most (95%) are due to Graves' disease which is an autoimmnune disorder caused by thyroid-stimulating hormone (TSH) receptor-stimulating antibodies.

More rarely, it may be due to toxic multinodular goitre or toxic adenoma, or occasionally subacute thyroiditis, iodine or lithium therapy.

- Diagnosis is established by finding a raised free T3 and free T4 and suppression of TSH.
- The clinical features of thyrotoxicosis can overlap with normal pregnancy particularly if there is a non-toxic goitre or anxiety.
- If a solitary nodule is present a fine needle biopsy should be considered to rule out malignancy.
- Carbimazole and propyl thiouracil are the most commonly used drugs. Most patients are treated for 12–18 months but the relapse rate is high and long-term treatment may be required. Though both drugs cross the placenta, propyl thiouracil does so less than carbimazole and thus should be the first choice for newly diagnosed women in pregnancy. The aim of treatment is to control the thyrotoxicosis as rapidly as possible and then maintain control with the lowest possible doses. Patients should be warned that the development of a sore throat or mouth ulcers necessitates the cessation of therapy and urgent medical attention because of the risk of agranulocytosis.
- Women should be seen monthly in the case of newly diagnosed cases but thyroid function tests are required less frequently in the case of those who are stable on antithyroid drugs.
- Beta-blockers can be used initially to improve the symptoms of tachycardia, sweating and tremors.
- Thyroidectomy is rarely required in pregnancy but if required may be safely performed in the second trimester. It is usually reserved for those with dysphagia or stridor related to a large goitre, those with suspected or confirmed carcinoma and those who have allergies to both antithyroid drugs.
- Radioiodine therapy is contraindicated in pregnancy and breastfeeding as it is taken up by the fetal thyroid with resulting thyroid ablation and hypothyroidism.
- Fetal or neonatal thyrotoxicosis occurs in 1–10% of babies with a past or current history of Graves' disease and may be predicted by measuring the level of thyroid-stimulating antibodies. Without treatment the mortality may reach 50% if the condition develops *in utero*. It may present with fetal tachycardia, intrauterine growth retardation or goitre. In the neonate the features include weight loss, tachycardia, irritability, jitteriness, poor feeding, goitre and congestive cardiac failure. Here, mortality is 15% without treatment.
- Serial ultrasound should be undertaken to check for growth, heart rate and fetal neck.

- In the case of fetal thyrotoxicosis, the mother is given antithyroid drugs, combined with thyroxine if she is euthyroid.
- The paediatricians should be made aware of treated cases.
- Breastfeeding is not contraindicated.

Q47. A 35-year-old woman at 26 weeks gestation presents with signs and symptoms consistent with pulmonary embolism. Critically appraise your management.

A47.

- Pulmonary thromboembolism (PTE) remains the major cause of maternal mortality in the UK. It is imperative that it is immediately recognized and treatment instituted as soon as possible in order to prevent mortality and morbidity.
- The treatment for pulmonary thromboembolism is prompt anticoagulation. In order to avoid the risks, inconvenience and cost of inappropriate anticoagulation, diagnostic imaging should be performed as soon as the diagnosis is suspected. If this is not immediately possible, anticoagulation should be started until an objective diagnosis is made.
- The diagnosis of PTE is confirmed by a ventilation perfusion scan. Treatment should be continued when the V/Q scan shows a medium to high probability of PTE. Bilateral leg Dopplers should simultaneously be carried out to rule out DVT.
- If clinical suspicion is high in spite of a negative V/Q scan and leg Dopplers, treatment should be continued and imaging repeated in a week. Pulmonary angiography, MRI or helical CT should be considered in these cases (if postpartum).
- D-dimers are not useful as a screening test as they may be elevated in pregnant women. A low level may however, suggest the absence of thromboembolism and thus may be useful.
- Initial therapy may include continuous intravenous infusion of unfractionated heparin, subcutaneous unfractionated heparin or subcutaneous low molecular weight heparin. In the former cases therapy is adjusted according to the APTT ratio which should be maintained between 1.5 and 2.5 times the average laboratory control value. LMWH is monitored by the anti-Xa levels.
- Mobilization with graduated elastic compression stockings should be encouraged.
- Women with recurrent PE may require a temporary caval filter. Surgical embolectomy and thrombolytic therapy should be considered.

- Maintenance treatment in the pregnant woman should be done with an adjusted dose regimen of subcutaneous unfractionated heparin or subcutaneous LMWH. In the postnatal period, oral anticoagulation with warfarin should be started and continued for at least 6–12 weeks. Warfarin is not contraindicated in breastfeeding.
- Heparin treatment should be continued until the INR on warfarin is between 2.0 and 3.0.
- The platelet count should be monitored on a monthly basis to look for thrombocytopaenia.
- The dose of heparin should be reduced to its thromboprophylactic dose on the day prior to induction or caesarean section. Regional anaesthesia should not be used at least 12 h after the previous prophylactic dose of LMWH.

Q48. A woman attending for a routine antenatal appointment complains of generalized itching. There is no sign of a rash or allergy and she is not on any medication. She is found to have mild jaundice and is 32 weeks into her pregnancy. Critically appraise your investigations and management.

A48.

- In the above case, in the absence of dermatoses and reaction to drugs or chemicals, a likely diagnosis is that of obstetric cholestasis. This is a liver disease of unknown aetiology that usually occurs in the latter half of pregnancy and is associated with generalized pruritis, abnormal liver function tests and raised bile acids.
- Liver function tests should be promptly carried out. These will reveal raised serum transaminases (two-to threefold) with raised bile acids.
- It is important to rule out other causes of liver disorders such as viral hepatitis, cholelithiasis, primary biliary cirrhosis and autoimmune chronic active hepatitis. With a view to doing this it may be necessary to carry out a liver ultrasound along with a serum hepatitis screen and antimitochondrial antibodies.
- There is a high perinatal mortality rate associated with the condition. Thus it is imperative that the fetus be monitored carefully with growth scans, biophysical profiles and Doppler umbilical artery velocimetry.
- In view of the fact that the condition is associated with late stillbirths, it is recommended that labour be induced around 37–38 weeks unless deteriorating liver functions or fetal condition warrants an earlier delivery.

- Ursodeoxycholic acid is associated with improvement in liver functions and pruritis and is a useful drug for this condition.
- With severe or prolonged cholestasis, deficiency of vitamin K may occur and supplements should be given to the mother before delivery and to the neonate.

Q49. A woman books in her first pregnancy at 6 weeks gestation. She suffers from sickle cell disease and wants to know the consequences of this on her pregnancy and on the fetus. She is married to her first cousin. Justify the counselling you would give her, and your management of her pregnancy.

A49.

- Sickle cell disease is an inherited disorder of haemoglobin synthesis. In sufferers it may cause a 'sickling' crisis precipitated by infection, dehydration, cold, hypoxia and pregnancy. This may result in infarction and pain. It is important to see these women early in pregnancy and explain the possible complications as well as explore the issues of prenatal testing and diagnosis.
- The partner should be tested for sickle cell disease or sickle cell trait (HbAS). If found to be positive or a carrier, prenatal diagnosis in the form of chorionic villus sampling, amniocentesis or cordocentesis should be offered.
- Antenatal care of the mother should involve a joint approach between a haematologist and obstetrician. The booking visit should involve testing for haemoglobin, blood group and antibodies, liver function tests, serology for syphilis, rubella, HIV, hepatitis B and C. Folic acid should be offered, though iron should not be given unless low ferritin levels indicate a coexisting iron deficiency.
- During pregnancy, these women should be warned that they are at an increased risk of sickle crisis, urinary tract infections, pyelonephritis and pneumonia. Urine should be routinely tested for culture and sensitivity and blood transfusions considered if they are anaemic and symptomatic.
- Patients should be admitted to hospital in a sickle crisis and given adequate hydration with intravenous fluids, antibiotics, warmth and adequate analgesia. Anticoagulation with heparin and TED stockings should be used in view of the increased risk of thrombosis.
- There is a higher perinatal mortality rate associated with sickle cell disease, mainly due to maternal complications leading to stillbirths or severe prematurity. There is also a higher risk of intrauterine growth restriction.

[handwritten notes:]

Crisis is
infn - UTI / PN / Pneu
3.

Stillbirth
IUGR
prematurity

1. Genetic   2. (a)
   PND .   Thrombosis

4. IP. / Postnatal.
   fetal cord blood

- Serial scans for fetal growth after 28 weeks gestation along with Doppler umbilical artery velocimetry and biophysical profiles should be done.
- During labour, patients should be kept warm and adequately hydrated. Blood should be cross-matched. Continuous fetal monitoring should be undertaken. Epidural anaesthesia is preferred over general anaesthesia as there is less risk of not maintaining oxygenation.
- Active management of the third stage should be undertaken to reduce blood loss.
- Fetal cord blood should be taken for electrophoresis and repeated at 3–6 months as β-globin variants are only seen in adult haemoglobin.
- Prophylactic antibiotics and heparin should be considered in the puerperium to combat the increased risk of thrombosis and infections.

Q50. You are asked to see a woman on the postnatal ward, who has delivered a baby by caesarean section 3 days ago and seems to be severely depressed. Critically appraise how you will manage this situation?

A50.

- Postnatal depression is usually divided into 'maternity blues' and non-psychotic postnatal depression 'proper'.
- The former is characterized by tearfulness, mild hypochondriasis, anxiety and irritability, with the symptoms typically peaking on the third to the fifth postpartum day. This needs to be distinguished from early onset, more severe depression. The latter has a prevalence of around 13% with the peak time of onset being 4–6 weeks.
- It is important to identify risk factors such as a past history of psychiatric disorder, mood disorder during the pregnancy, poor marital relationship and lack of social support. Health-care workers should be well aware of this entity and able to assess the mother's mood, elucidate depressive symptoms and suicidal thoughts and arrange for appropriate professional psychiatric help if necessary.
- Antidepressants such as tricyclic antidepressants and selective serotonin uptake inhibitors such as fluoxetine can be used. Though they are secreted in breast milk, plasma concentrations in breast-fed infants are rarely detectable.
- There is no evidence to show that progestogens are effective for the treatment of postnatal depression.
- Any remediable social factors should be attended to including helping the partner in understanding the mother's need for emotional support, rest and practical help with the baby.

- The mother should be put in touch at discharge with local and national support groups such as the National Childbirth Trust, the Association for Postnatal Illness and the 'Meet a Mum' association.
- It is important to gauge if there is any risk to the baby or other children by the mother and involve psychiatrists and social workers as necessary.

Q51. A woman whose first child suffers from β-thalassaemia is now 8 weeks into her second pregnancy. She is very worried about the baby and comes to you for advice. No one else is affected in her immediate family. Justify the advice and counselling you will impart to her.

A51.
- It is imperative to give the woman an idea of the risk of recurrence of the condition. As thalassaemia is an autosomal recessive disorder, this is likely to be 1 : 4 if both partners are carriers.
- Prenatal diagnosis in the form of chorionic villus biopsy or fetal blood sampling is the method of choice to diagnose the condition and allow termination of an affected fetus. This allows for DNA analysis of fetal chromosomes.
- As CVS allows for more rapid and earlier diagnosis thus allowing early termination, this is the preferred method of diagnosis of the condition. However, it is associated with a miscarriage rate of 1 : 50.
- The other risks with CVS are that of an erroneous result due to placental mosaicisim which can occur in up to 1% of cases. In this case the woman will have to be prewarned of the need for an amniocentesis to confirm the result.
- It is important to counsel both partners together and to put them in touch with support groups for thalassaemia.

Q52. A 32-year-old woman at 20 weeks in her first pregnancy undergoes colposcopic examination for postcoital bleeding. She is found to have a growth on her cervix, which is later clinically staged to be a IIIb squamous cell carcinoma. Critically appraise your subsequent management.

A52.
- The incidence of invasive cervical cancer in pregnancy is around 1 in 1000 deliveries. Treatment of these cancers are based on the same principles as in non-pregnant patients with the exception that multiple factors have to be taken into consideration such as tumour size and stage, gestational age and the patient's own choice. In the case of early stage disease treatment may be delayed till fetal viability is reached.

- In this case, because of the advanced stage of the disease it is advisable to treat the patient as soon as possible. As she is still very early in gestation this would inevitably mean termination of the pregnancy.
- The treatment of choice in this case would be radiotherapy, both external beam radiation and brachytherapy.
- Most pregnancies would abort after external beam therapy. However, the choice of medical termination before radiation should be offered along with feticide.
- In case, after counselling, the woman decides she does not want a termination in order for treatment to be started, one should wait for fetal viability. This would usually be taken as 28 weeks. Steroids should be given at 27 weeks in order to promote fetal lung maturity and a caesarean section undertaken a week later.
- Treatment should then be planned with the oncologists. It is important that a multidisciplinary team consisting of the obstetricians, midwives, Macmillan nurses, gynaecological and medical oncologists, paediatricians and counsellors should be involved from the very beginning.

Q53. A 28-year-old woman who has been treated for breast cancer a year ago, comes to you for advice. She does not have any children and is very keen on starting a family. She has had adjuvant chemotherapy and is currently on tamoxifen. Critically appraise the advice you will impart to her.

A53.

- Breast cancer is the most common cancer amongst women and is the single commonest cause of deaths in women aged 35–54. Around 15% of breast cancers are seen in women of childbearing age, and as more and more women are delaying having children, pregnancy in women with a history of breast cancer is becoming commoner.
- It is important to advise the woman in the context of a multidisciplinary team comprising the clinical oncologist, surgeon and obstetrician. A full history of the disease should be available, including stage at diagnosis, treatment and follow-up including recurrence or remission.
- A third of women under 40 years of age, who undergo chemotherapy for breast cancer will develop amenorrhoea and anovulation. However, this is usually temporary. As long as ovulation and menstruation are resumed, reassurances about fertility can be given to the woman.
- Pregnancy in women under 33–35 years of age should be delayed for about 2–3 years. This is to reduce the risk of relapse and also to differentiate

those with a better prognosis for long-term survival from those with more aggressive disease.

- Adjuvant chemotherapy and radiotherapy do not have any ill effects upon a subsequent pregnancy or the fetus.
- Contraception should be advised while the woman is on tamoxifen as this may lead to spontaneous abortions, birth defects and fetal death. Similarly, tamoxifen should not be taken in pregnancy.
- Where possible, there is no contraindication for breastfeeding.
- The woman can be reassured that unless there is a genetic predisposition to cancers, children of survivors of breast cancer do not have an increased incidence of birth defects or childhood cancer.

Q54. A 27-year-old woman has recently undergone a renal transplantation and is contemplating a pregnancy. What advice, specific to her condition would you give her?

A54.

- Women who have undergone a renal transplantation are usually advised to wait a year or two before getting pregnant. The reason for this is that by this time they are usually at maintenance levels (minimum dose) of immunosuppressives. Also, if renal functions are normal at this stage, they have an 80% 5-year survival rate.
- It is important to stress that good pregnancy outcomes of around 90% occur in women with normal preconceptual renal functions. This goes down to 70% however, if pregnancy complications occur before 28 weeks.
- There is an increased incidence of early and late pregnancy loss in these women.
- If the patient is on ACE inhibitors, they will need to be changed to β-blockers.
- There are risks involved as complications such as hypertension and pre-eclampsia (30%), graft rejection (10%), intrauterine growth retardation (20–40%) and preterm labour (40–60%) may develop. This warrants a close monitoring of the pregnancy and fetus with frequent renal function tests, growth scans and umbilical artery doppler measurements.
- Most renal grafts function very well in pregnancy. There is a higher incidence however, of proteinuria (40%), and urinary tract infections. In 15% of cases, renal complications may persist after delivery.
- The other important point to make to the patient is the safety of immunosuppressive drugs that she is on. This is because reduction or cessation of these drugs may cause graft rejection.

1. wait Conf. 2-3 y. - renal fn.
2. 90% ℗ - ℗ devolfn.
3. ACE inhi
4. Immunos - cont.
5. Comp

HTN/ PE, infn. RN, Graft reju.

Baby Early, Late loss
IUGR
Preterm .

Prednisolone, azathioprine and cyclosporin A are the main drugs used. Prednisolone can cause glucose intolerance, hence testing for diabetes is indicated. Cyclosporin can be nephrotoxic and is associated with hypertension and intrauterine growth retardation. Serum levels need to be monitored. These drugs are safe with breastfeeding.

- Labour and delivery in renal transplant patients is not very different from other women. Caesareans are done only for obstetric indications. The graft does not interfere with normal labour.
- Steroid cover is needed for labour and delivery, and prophylactic antibiotics are needed for operative procedures.

Q55. A 36-year-old woman who is pregnant for the first time is a severe asthmatic. What particular precautions will you take while managing her pregnancy?

A55.

- Asthma is a common chronic medical condition that affects pregnant women, with 3–5% of women suffering from it in pregnancy. It exacerbates in around one-third of women in pregnancy, and a similar proportion improve or remain unchanged. Asthma severity usually returns to prepregnancy levels within 3 months of delivery.
- Though in most women there are no adverse effects of asthma on pregnancy outcome, in poorly controlled asthmatics, chronic maternal hypoxaemia may adversely affect the fetus.
- There is an association with pregnancy-induced hypertension and pre-eclampsia, as well as preterm birth, low birth weight and neonatal morbidity in the form of transient tachypnoea of the newborn, hypoglycaemia and neonatal seizures.
- Objective assessments in the form of pulmonary function tests and frequent home monitoring with peak flow measurements should be recommended.
- It is important to reassure women about the safety of medication including β_2-agonists, inhaled and systemic corticosteroids in pregnancy as well as lactation.
- Acute, severe attacks should be aggressively managed in hospital. These women need intravenous hydration, oxygen and nebulizers of β_2-agonists. A chest X-ray should be performed to exclude pneumonia or pneumothorax. Intravenous and oral steroids may be needed along with intravenous aminophylline. Steroids should be tapered on discharge, with a review appointment with a chest physician arranged.

PIH   LBW   PFT
PE   TTN   Home
               Seizures   admit
                              PGF2α

- Women receiving oral steroids should get intravenous hydrocortisone three to four times a day during labour until oral medication is restarted.
- It is important to bear in mind bronchospasm caused by the administration of prostaglandin $F_{2\alpha}$, used for postpartum haemorrhage, though $PGE_{2\alpha}$ used for induction of labour is a bronchodilater and is safe.
- All forms of analgesia in labour including epidural analgesia and entonox are safe. In case of severe acute attacks during labour, epidural anaesthesia is preferred due to the reduced risk of pneumonia and atelectasis.

Q56. 'Low molecular weight heparins are better than conventional heparin in the prevention and treatment of thromboembolic episodes'. Justify this statement.
A56.

- Low molecular weight (LMW) heparins are fragments of conventional heparin produced by enzymatic and chemical breakdown. Conventional heparin has mainly two actions, it acts in tandem with antithrombin III, to which it attaches, and has an inhibitory action on Xa and IIa.
- Because of their shorter structure, LMWHs contain the antithrombin binding site for action against Xa, but do not possess the region necessary to inhibit IIa. Therefore they have a predominantly antithrombotic effect, without having anticoagulant activity.
- There is a lower risk of haemorrhagic complications. There is also minimal alteration in thrombin time and activated partial thromboplastin time. Thus frequent blood tests to check these parameters are not needed.
- They are associated with a lower risk of thrombocytopaenia. They have increased bioavailability and a longer half-life, thus once daily administration is sufficient. As therapy may be needed for long periods, this means better compliance and patient acceptability.
- They may be associated with less bone loss, though this aspect is still being researched.

Q57. A patient is referred to you at 26 weeks gestation. She has recently come to the UK from abroad and has been diagnosed to be suffering from pulmonary tuberculosis. Evaluate your management plan.
A57.

- The incidence of women suffering from tuberculosis in the UK is increasing due to the rising immigrant population as well as a higher incidence of the condition associated with HIV infection. Tuberculosis does not

Sputum for AFB
Chest X ray - RUL
Bronchial - pul. aspirates
Mantoux
Heaf

have a detrimental effect on pregnancy as long as prompt and effective treatment is administered.

- It is important to bear in mind that untreated tuberculosis presents a greater hazard to women and their fetuses than the treatment itself. The advice of a respiratory physician should always be sought before embarking on treatment.
- Antituberculous treatment mainly consists of triple or quadruple therapy with rifampicin, isoniazid, pyrazinamide and/or ethambutol.
- Ethambutol and isoniazid are safe to use in pregnancy, but all patients taking isoniazid should also be prescribed pyridoxine 50 mg/day to reduce the risk of peripheral neuritis.
- Streptomycin has been associated with a high incidence of VIIIth nerve damage and should be avoided in pregnancy. There are no proven adverse effects on the fetus with rifampicin.
- Pyrazinamide is best avoided during organogenesis because of paucity of safety data.
- Liver function tests should be monitored regularly. The patient should be nursed in isolation in the beginning. She will usually become non-infectious within 2 weeks of starting treatment.
- The neonate should be given the BCG vaccination at birth, and prophylactic treatment with isoniazid in case the mother is sputum positive.
- Though antituberculosis drugs are excreted in breast milk, they do so in minute quantities, and breastfeeding is safe.

Public health issue, Contact tracing Social issue

Q58. Critically appraise the use of anticoagulants in pregnant women with prosthetic heart valves.

A58.

- There is a need to maintain a high level of anticoagulation in women with prosthetic heart valves because of the risk of thromboembolic complications. This is especially true for mechanical prosthetic heart valves as compared to bioprosthetic or homograft valves.
- Though heparin is safe from the fetal point of view as it does not cross the placenta, it is associated with a greater risk of thromboembolic complications. It is also associated with osteoporosis and thrombocytopaenia when used long term.
- Warfarin is teratogenic and causes an embryopathy characterized by stippled epiphysis and nasal hypoplasia, particularly if exposed between 6 and 12 weeks gestation. This risk can be eliminated by using heparin between the 6–12th weeks of gestation. The use of warfarin in the second and third trimesters is associated with central nervous system defects such

as Dandy–Walker malformation, midline cerebellar atrophy and optic atrophy.

- Women should be thoroughly counselled regarding the risks of anti-coagulant use in pregnancy on the one hand, and the absolute necessity for it on the other. An informed decision needs to be taken at the beginning of the pregnancy regarding the choice of anticoagulation.

- The optimal regimen consists of warfarin used throughout pregnancy, with heparin substituted between 6 and 12 weeks. Close monitoring of anticoagulation treatment is mandatory, with an INR of 2.5–3.5 for women on warfarin, and an APTT ratio of 2.0–2.5 for women on heparin. Low molecular weight heparin is usually preferred because of the need for less frequent administration and more predictable side-effect profile. Anti-Xa assay is used for monitoring.

- Only heparin should be given from 36 weeks onwards to allow time for the reversal of the anticoagulant effect of warfarin because of the imma-turity of the fetal liver, thereby reducing the risk of cerebral haemorrhage. Heparin is stopped at the time of delivery and recommenced soon afterwards using intravenous heparin initially and then warfarin. They are both safe for use while breastfeeding.

Q59. One week after a normal delivery, a previously healthy woman starts complaining of breathlessness and chest pain. She has an echocardiogram, suggesting the diagnosis of cardiomyopathy. Outline the principles of management.

A59.

- Peripartum cardiomyopathy occurs in relation to pregnancy in women with no prior history of heart disease. There is usually development of cardiac failure in relation to left ventricular dysfunction. There is no proven cause of the condition, though myocarditis, abnormal immune response, and a greater susceptibility to viral infections due to suppressed cell-mediated immunity have all been proposed.

- It is associated with a high mortality rate of 25–50% with death being mainly due to cardiac failure, arrhythmias or thromboembolic complications.

- Cardiac failure is treated with diuretics, digoxin and vasodilators.

- Angiotensin-converting enzyme inhibitors can be used postnatally, though they are contraindicated in the pregnant patient due to terato-genecity in the form of fetal renal defects when used in the second and third trimesters. Hydralazine is a safe and useful after-load reducing agent.

Cardiac failure.
arrythmia
Thromboembolism
Supp.
Med   Ig
Self-card. Transplant
Medical disorders in pregnancy 75
Flu.

- Thromboembolic complications are common and anticoagulation should be used in those with a significantly reduced left ventricular ejection fraction or cardiac arrhythmias. Heparin and warfarin can both be used safely after delivery.
- If the patient fails to respond within 2 weeks of supportive therapy, intravenous immunoglobulin may be useful.
- Cardiac transplantation is a final option for those who continue to deteriorate or fail to respond to medical treatment.
- In case of persistent left ventricular dysfunction 6 months after delivery, women should be strongly advised against attempting another pregnancy.

Q60. A woman suffering from systemic lupus nephritis wishes to start a family. Critically appraise the advice you will give her and your proposed management of her pregnancy.

A60.

- Systemic lupus erythematosus is a systemic connective tissue disease associated with periods of disease activity called 'flares' and of remissions.
- The woman should be advised to get pregnant during the period of remission. Though renal functions are not affected in the long term, pregnancy in women with lupus nephritis is associated with an increased incidence of fetal loss, pre-eclampsia and intrauterine growth retardation. The prognosis is associated with serum creatinine levels, with a level above 132 μmol/L being associated with a 50% fetal loss rate.
- The pregnancy should be managed jointly by both the physicians and obstetricians, thus ensuring that disease activity is monitored along with the fetal condition.
- Azathioprine is commonly used to control the condition and is safe. Non-steroidal anti-inflammatory agents are not teratogenic, though if used in the third trimester, may be associated with premature closure of the ductus arteriosus in the fetus. The woman should be reassured about the safety of prednisolone, and the importance of complying with her medication. Hydrochloroquine should be continued, as stopping it may precipitate a flare. Cyclophosphamide is contraindicated.
- Hypertension is usually treated with methyldopa.
- It is difficult to distinguish between pre-eclampsia and lupus nephritis in pregnancy as they both have similar symptoms. Though a renal biopsy is a means of definitive diagnosis, it is seldom carried out. A rising anti-DNA titre and the presence of red blood cells or casts in the urine may

indicate lupus nephritis. Early delivery may be warranted in case of worsening pre-eclampsia.

- Fetal monitoring in the form of growth scans, uterine artery and umbilical artery Doppler blood flow measurements should be routinely carried out.
- The woman should be warned of the risk of congenital heart block in the fetus in the presence of anti-Ro antibodies. This is present in 2–5% of babies of Ro-positive mothers. Another phenomenon is the development of neonatal cutaneous lupus in 5% of these children.

Chapter 3
Obstetric emergencies

Chapter 3: Questions

Answers are on pp. 80–97

Q61. A 28-week pregnant woman is admitted with epigastric pain. Her blood pressure is 160/120 and she has 3+ proteinuria. Liver function tests reveal AST of 100 U/L, serum urates are elevated, and the platelet count is 56 000/µL. Justify your subsequent management.

Q62. A woman is brought to hospital via an ambulance. She has bled vaginally profusely and is unconscious and according to the paramedics is around 9 months pregnant. Justify your initial management.

Q63. A pregnant woman at 37 weeks is admitted with abdominal pain and vaginal bleeding. She is found to have a tense and tender abdomen. Ultrasound scan reveals a normally situated placenta but no fetal heart is seen on scan. Justify your subsequent management.

Q64. A 38-year-old woman presents in established labour at term in her second pregnancy. In the past she had a caesarean section for breech presentation. Two subsequent examinations reveal no progress in cervical dilatation and an oxytocin drip is started. Two hours later she complains of severe abdominal pain in spite of an epidural. The cardiotocograph reveals reduced variability with late decelerations. You are the labour ward registrar and are called to see her. Justify the principles of your management.

Q65. A woman undergoes a scan at 34 weeks gestation, which reveals a low-lying anterior placenta covering the internal os. She is in her third pregnancy having had two previous caesarean sections. An elective caesarean section at 39 weeks reveals an abnormally adherent placenta. Justify your management.

Q66. You are called urgently to see a patient who had a normal vaginal delivery 15 min ago followed by a brisk vaginal blood loss. This was followed by a drop in blood pressure and the midwife noticed the uterus inverted at the introitus with the placenta still attached. Describe the steps you will take in this situation.

Q67. A woman is treated for postpartum haemorrhage on the high dependency unit. She is then found to be oliguric with rising urea and creatinine levels. Critically appraise the principles of management of this emergency.

Q68. You are the registrar on call for labour ward and are called urgently by the SHO who has just conducted a forceps delivery. On arrival you find the woman in lithotomy position with a steady trickle of blood, extensive tears to the vulva, vagina and periurethral areas, and a possible third degree tear. She is haemodynamically stable, and the SHO has managed to insert two wide bore intravenous needles and has sent off blood for cross-matching. Critically appraise your management.

Q69. You are the senior registrar on call for labour ward and are crash called to a delivery room. On entering you find the registrar dealing with a shoulder dystocia. He has already tried the McRobert's manoeuvre along with suprapubic pressure without success. It has been 4 min since the delivery of the head. Detail the steps you will take.

Q70. Critically appraise the role of risk management in shoulder dystocia.

Q71. A woman presents at 28 weeks gestation complaining of severe right-sided abdominal pain, nausea, vomiting and fever. Critically appraise how you will go about reaching a diagnosis and instituting management.

Q72. You are the on-call registrar when you are crash called to attend to a woman brought in to casualty after a major road traffic accident. She is unconscious, with shallow respiration, and is bleeding from multiple wounds. She is also 30 weeks pregnant. Justify your management.

Q73. You are called urgently to see a woman who delivered a baby 2 h ago and subsequently complains of sudden chills, sweating, breathlessness followed by shock, cyanosis and cardiovascular collapse. Critically appraise your management.

Q74. A woman has her first eclamptic fit immediately after delivery in hospital. What principles underlie her subsequent management?

Q75. A 32-year-old primiparous woman at 34 weeks gestation is admitted with a blood pressure of 140/90 mmHg and 2+ proteinuria. She starts complaining of severe epigastric pain, nausea and vomiting. Serum biochemical values are as follows: aspartate transaminase 100 μmol/L, urates 600 μmol/L, plasma glucose 1.4 mmol/L, platelets 75 × 10^9/L. Critically appraise how you will reach a diagnosis and manage the case.

Q76. You are asked to see a woman suffering from puerperial pyrexia. Outline your management.

Q77. A midwife calls you urgently to a normal delivery, which has just occurred. The baby is pale and gasping. You know the paediatrician is currently in theatre attending a caesarian section. Describe your actions clearly.

Q78. You are called upon to urgently review a woman who had a normal delivery 40 min ago. Following this she started trickling blood vaginally. Initial measures taken by the midwife have not halted the bleeding. Those included starting an oxytocin infusion intravenously and inspecting the perineum which appears to be intact. The placenta and membranes have also been inspected and appear complete. The woman continues to bleed and the estimated blood loss by now is around 900 mL. Critically appraise the steps you will take to manage this emergency.

Q79. 'Domestic violence often goes unnoticed and unreported.' Critically appraise how you will recognize signs of an abusive relationship and what steps you would take to help the victim of such abuse, with particular reference to the antenatal period.

Chapter 3: **Answers**

Q61. A 28-week pregnant woman is admitted with epigastric pain. Her blood pressure is 160/120 and she has 3+ proteinuria. Liver function tests reveal AST of 100 U/L, serum urates are elevated, and the platelet count is 56 000/μL. Justify your management.

A61.

- The picture with which the above patient has presented suggests the diagnosis of severe pre-eclampsia with the superimposition of HELLP syndrome. This is a severe and life-threatening condition which needs to be dealt with expeditiously in order to prevent maternal and fetal morbidity and mortality.
- The priority is to stabilize maternal condition. This is done by administering antihypertensives to bring down the blood pressure to avoid cerebrovascular accidents. A choice of intravenous hydralazine or labetalol can be used.
- The patient needs to be cared for on the high dependency unit of a tertiary referral centre with a multidisciplinary team consisting of senior obstetric, anaesthetic, paediatric and haematological staff involved.
- Haemolysis should be looked for on a blood smear with the presence of Burr cells, schistocytes and elevated lactate dehydrogenase. Frequent monitoring of biochemical parameters should be done. Worsening of the condition is suggested by increasing transaminases and falling platelets. Coagulation status should be checked, as disseminated intravascular coagulation (DIC) is often a feature. DIC should be aggressively treated with fresh frozen plasma.
- In case platelets fall below 20 000/μL, platelet transfusions should be considered.
- It is important to look for fetal well-being in the form of growth scan, Doppler umbilical blood flow velocimetries and biophysical profiles.
- Steroids should be administered to the mother for fetal lung maturity in case prompt delivery is required.
- Once maternal condition is stabilized, a decision regarding expediting delivery should be made. This would usually be by caesarean section.
- Epidural anaesthesia is contraindicated due to thrombocytopaenia.
- Once delivered, the patient should undergo intensive monitoring on the intensive care unit. The risk of pulmonary oedema and ARDS should be recognized and a strict monitoring of fluid balance should be done, preferably with the aid of central venous pressure or Swan–Ganz monitoring.

Q62. A woman is brought to hospital via an ambulance. She has had profuse vaginal bleeding and is unconscious and according to the paramedics is around 9 months pregnant. Justify your initial management.

A62.

- The first and foremost objective in this case is to resuscitate the patient. The principles of this are to check airway, breathing and circulation (A, B, C).
- An intravenous line with a wide bore cannula (size 14–16 gauge) must immediately be inserted if not done so already.
- Blood should be obtained at the same time for a full blood count, cross-matching, urea and electrolytes and a coagulation profile. Six units of blood should immediately be ordered for cross-matching.
- Intravenous fluids should be given while awaiting blood. This should be in the form of colloids. Consideration should be given to transfusing O rhesus negative blood if there is a delay in cross-matching. However this should only be transfused if it is lifesaving.
- Senior help should be immediately sought. Both the obstetric and anaesthetic consultants and the theatre team should be immediately informed and assembled.
- Once maternal condition is stable, checking the fetal condition must be done by listening to the fetal heart. This is accompanied by a quick scan to look for placental position.
- In case of placenta praevia a caesarean section is indicated regardless of fetal condition.
- In case of placental abruption, caesarean section is indicated with a live fetus. In case of IUD, vaginal delivery after induction of labour should be attempted.

Q63. A pregnant woman at 37 weeks is admitted with abdominal pain and vaginal bleeding. She is found to have a tense and tender abdomen. Ultrasound scan reveals a normally situated placenta but no fetal heart is seen on scan. Justify your subsequent management.

A63.

- The diagnosis in this case is most likely of a severe placental abruption.
- Coagulopathy is one of the real risks with severe placental abruption and this must be looked for by doing a coagulation profile including fibrinogen levels, fibrin degradation products (FDP), PT, PTT, thrombin time and a platelet count.

- As the fetus is dead, vaginal delivery is the goal. This can be undertaken by artificial rupture of the membranes followed by intravenous oxytocin.
- Only if maternal shock is incorrectable or if there is an obstetric indication such as a transverse lie, should a caesarean section be undertaken.
- Adequate analgesia should be provided though in case of severe haemorrhage with disseminated intravascular coagulation(DIC) an epidural is contraindicated.
- Initial management of a coagulopathy is the replacement of blood volume and consumed clotting factors. This is done by administering fresh frozen plasma, fibrinogen or platelets as required. However, the ultimate treatment of DIC is delivery of the fetus and placenta.

Q64. A 38-year-old woman presents in established labour at term in her second pregnancy. In the past she had a caesarean section for breech presentation. Two subsequent examinations reveal no progress in cervical dilatation and an oxytocin drip is started. Two hours later she complains of severe abdominal pain, particularly at the site of the uterine scar in spite of an epidural. The cardiotocograph reveals reduced variability with late decelerations. You are the labour ward registrar and are called to see her. Justify the principles of your management.

A64.

- The most likely diagnosis in this case is a uterine rupture. The most common cause for this is a previous caesarean section scar. A previous classical scar confers a 3–4% rupture rate. A lower segment scar however, confers a 0.25–0.50% rate of scar rupture.
- Other signs to confirm the diagnosis include bleeding, fetal parts palpable outside the uterus, and a fetal head, which retracts back up the maternal abdomen.
- It is important to take swift action if the lives of the mother and baby are to be saved. Senior obstetric and anaesthetic help should immediately be summoned and the woman transferred to theatre.
- Large bore intravenous access should be ensured and blood sent off for cross-matching. An immediate laparotomy should be undertaken and senior obstetric help summoned. Also, senior paediatric help to resuscitate the baby should be available.
- In case of a stable patient with an uncomplicated rupture, surgical repair of the rupture site is acceptable. In this case it is advisable to perform an elective caesarean section in the next pregnancy at 36 weeks.
- In many cases, caesarean hysterectomy is necessary to control bleeding.

- An important aspect of management is proper postnatal counselling and explanation of events as often there is no time for detailed discussions at the time of the emergency and this often leaves patients unsatisfied. This should be undertaken by the consultant in charge of the woman's care.

Q65. A woman undergoes a scan at 34 weeks gestation, which reveals a low-lying anterior placenta covering the internal os. She is in her third pregnancy having had two previous caesarean sections. An elective caesarean section at 39 weeks reveals an abnormally adherent placenta. Justify your management.

A65.

- Placenta accreta is the abnormal adherence of the placenta wholly or partly to the uterine wall. It may be placenta increta, where it invades deeply into the myometrium or placenta percreta, where the placenta penetrates the uterine serosa.
- There is a high incidence of placenta accreta with a low-lying placenta in patients with previous caesarean sections. This is due to adherence of the placenta to the previous uterine scar. This fact should have been anticipated before elective caesarean delivery in this case and proper counselling regarding the risks involved with consent for a caesarean hysterectomy taken beforehand.
- Delivery in this case should be conducted by a senior obstetrician with the involvement of senior anaesthetic staff.
- Blood should be cross-matched and other blood products such as fresh frozen plasma should be readily available if needed. The consultant haematologist should be informed.
- If the patient is stable and haemorrhage under control then conservative measures such as over-sewing the implantation site or uterine artery ligation may be attempted.
- If the haemorrhage is uncontrollable, the treatment of choice is a hysterectomy.
- Leaving the placenta *in situ* is not an option because of the risk of haemorrhage and infection.

Q66. You are called urgently to see a patient who had a normal vaginal delivery 15 min ago followed by a brisk vaginal blood loss. This was followed by a drop in blood pressure and the midwife noticed the uterus inverted at the introitus with the placenta still attached. Describe the steps you will take in this situation.

A66.

- Uterine inversion occurs in around 1 in 2000 deliveries and is associated with haemorrhage in a majority of cases and is often associated with shock. The uterus is often found protruding from the vagina but where it does not do so it may go undetected and result in a subacute or chronic inversion.
- The treatment of hypovolaemia and shock is the first priority and large bore venous access should be secured, intravenous fluids started with blood sent off for cross-matching and clotting screen. Appropriate senior obstetric and anaesthetic help should be summoned.
- An attempt should be made to reposition the uterus in the vagina without removing the placenta. The sooner this is done the greater chances of success.
- If manual reposition is unsuccessful, uterine relaxants such as intravenous ritodrine or terbutaline are used. After successful replacement of the uterus manual removal of the placenta is performed. Once the uterus is in position the attendant's hand should remain in the endometrial cavity until a firm contraction occurs with intravenous oxytocin.
- If the above method is unsuccessful, O'Sullivan's technique of hydrostatic replacement is tried. Two litres of saline are placed on an intravenous stand and kept approximately 2 m above the ground. The introitus is manually sealed while sterile fluid is instilled into the vagina. A silastic vacuum cup can be used to accomplish a seal.
- If all methods fail, abdominal correction of uterine inversion via a laparotomy is carried out by either the Huntington or Haltain procedures.

Q67. A woman is treated for postpartum haemorrhage on the high dependency unit. She is then found to be oliguric with rising urea and creatinine levels. Critically appraise the principles of management of this emergency.

A67.

- In this case the likely diagnosis is the onset of acute renal failure. The serum urea usually rises to a much higher level than the creatinine. A senior renal physician should be involved at an early stage in the treatment of this woman.
- The signs of acute renal failure should be looked for. These are hypertension, renal angle tenderness, signs of pulmonary oedema, and acidotic breathing.

- The diagnosis should be confirmed by investigations, which include serial blood urea and creatinine, serum electrolytes, and urine microscopy to rule out acute tubular necrosis.
- A renal ultrasound is helpful in delineating any obstruction to the kidneys.
- A central venous line should be sited if not present already, to give an accurate estimate of the intravascular volume status.
- The cornerstone of treatment is the restoration of intravascular volume. A strict input–output fluid chart is mandatory. Excessive blood losses should be replaced by blood products and crystalloids used for maintenance. Fluid balance is particularly crucial in cases of pre-eclampsia. Potassium-containing fluid should be avoided as it will compound the problem of hyperkalaemia.
- Loop diuretics such as frusemide are used to increase urine output and to treat pulmonary oedema if present.
- Serum electrolytes should be regularly checked to look for signs of hyperkalaemia and hyponatraemia. Metabolic acidosis is the other feature to look for and is corrected by giving bicarbonate.
- Drugs that may aggravate the condition should be stopped. These include non-steroidal anti-inflammatory agents and aminoglycosides.
- In case of the onset of complications, dialysis may be needed until the kidneys recover.

Q68. You are the registrar on call for labour ward and are called urgently by the SHO who has just conducted a forceps delivery. On arrival you find the woman in lithotomy position with a steady trickle of blood, extensive tears to the vulva, vagina and periurethral areas, and a possible third degree tear. She is haemodynamically stable, and the SHO has managed to insert two wide bore intravenous needles and has sent off blood for cross-matching. Critically appraise your management.
A68.

- In such a case of extensive perineal trauma following an instrumental delivery where active bleeding is taking place, prompt action and the early involvement of senior assistance is mandatory.
- After the primary management to ensure intravenous fluid replacement and the prompt cross-matching of blood, the patient should be transferred to the operating theatre for a detailed examination under anaesthesia and repair. This will ensure adequate analgesia and good lighting which are essential.

- Blood should be replaced as soon as it is available. The haematology laboratory as well as the consultant should be informed.
- A detailed examination under anaesthesia should be carried out to identify injured structures. Any bleeding cervical lacerations should be repaired carefully, taking care not to inadvertently insert sutures into the bladder (anterior tears), or the ureter (posterior tears).
- Vaginal lacerations should be sutured, and if oozing from multiple lacerations continue, a tight vaginal pack is inserted for 24 h. A urethral catheter should be inserted to avoid urinary retention. This is also useful in delineating the urethra while suturing any paraurethral tears.
- Any haematoma should be surgically explored. Infralevator haematomas require insertion of deep sutures at their base. Supralevator haematomas may form in the broad ligament due to extension of cervical or vaginal tears and are conservatively managed.
- Careful exploration of the anal sphincter and mucosa will reveal any third or fourth degree tears. In the latter, the torn anal epithelium is sutured with interrupted 3–0 Vicryl sutures, with the knots tied in the anal lumen. The internal anal sphincter should be identified, and any tears sutured separately from the external anal sphincter with interrupted 3–0 PDS. The external anal sphincter should also be repaired by 3–0 PDS, with the use of either the overlapping or end-to-end method. A stool softener such as lactulose should be prescribed along with antibiotics.

Q69. You are the senior registrar on call for labour ward and are crash called to a delivery room. On entering you find the registrar dealing with a shoulder dystocia. He has already tried the McRobert's manoeuvre along with suprapubic pressure without success. It has been 4 min since the delivery of the head. Detail the steps you will take.
A69.
- The incidence of shoulder dystocia is around 1.2% of all deliveries, though only 10% will not respond to the measures listed above.
- It should be ensured that the consultant obstetrician, paediatrician and anaesthetist have been summoned.
- The 'Wood's screw manoeuvre' should be attempted. This entails inserting a hand in the vagina and applying digital pressure to the front aspect of the posterior shoulder, aided by continued suprapubic pressure. The entire trunk is rotated by 180 degrees around the long axis of the fetus. The anterior shoulder is brought off the pubic symphysis and the posterior is delivered from its new anterior position.

- Alternatively, delivery of the posterior arm is attempted by passing a hand into the vagina as far as the elbow of the posterior arm. The arm is flexed at the elbow and the wrist is grasped and traction applied to sweep the arm across the abdomen and chest. This arm is then delivered and the fetus rotated through 180 degrees. The other arm (which was previously lying anteriorly) is then delivered similarly from its new posterior position.
- If all the above manoeuvres have failed, a symphysiotomy or cleidotomy should be attempted.
- Cephalic replacement followed by a caesarean section (Zaveanelli manoeuvre) has been described, though experience is limited and it is tried only as a last resort.
- Meticulous notes of all the steps taken along with the times should be made and signed legibly.

Q70. Critically appraise the role of risk management in shoulder dystocia.

A70.

- Risk management as related to the occurrence of shoulder dystocia is aimed at predicting the occurrence beforehand and preventing it if possible.
- Risk factors associated with shoulder dystocia are macrosomia, diabetes mellitus and previous shoulder dystocia. However, as the sensitivity of any of the risk factors in preventing shoulder dystocia is poor, they cannot be the basis for offering these women elective caesarean delivery with all its inherent risks. The ability to predict fetal weight on the basis of scan or clinical judgement is poor, added to which a large number of cases occur in babies weighing less than 4 kg.
- It is vital that all labour ward staff are well versed in the manoeuvres to deal with shoulder dystocia and that guidelines are circulated and regularly updated. Regular 'drills' should be undertaken on delivery suite, teaching the manoeuvres to the staff.
- Where a risk factor is discovered antenatally, it should be communicated to the staff looking after the woman in labour. This can be done by highlighting it on the hand-held notes as well as requesting a registrar to be present at delivery on the labour pages of the case records.
- After the occurrence of the event, a full explanation should be given to the patient and her partner about what went on and why.

- Meticulous documentation of events, with dates, times and manoeuvres used, in what order and whether they were successful or not should be done. All entries should be legibly signed and records of any communications with patients should be kept.

Q71. A woman presents at 28 weeks gestation complaining of severe right-sided abdominal pain, nausea, vomiting and fever. Critically appraise how you will go about reaching a diagnosis and instituting management.

A71.

- Abdominal pain in pregnancy poses a peculiar diagnostic problem due to the anatomical and physiological changes which go with it. There is a risk of delayed diagnosis and hence a worse outcome, and therefore it is important to rule out the major causes.
- A detailed history of onset of pain, duration, radiation, aggravating and relieving factors must be taken. Uterine causes of severe acute onset pain are torsion of an ovarian cyst, and a degenerating fibroid. There may be a history of these conditions and an ultrasound scan may be able to detect them. Treatment is mainly conservative, in the form of bed rest and analgesia.
- Placental abruption occurs in approximately 0.5–1% of pregnancies. Although usually associated with visible vaginal bleeding, concealed accidental haemorrhage may occur where blood loss is mainly retroplacental. It is usually associated with fetal cardiotocograph abnormalities, and delivery should be considered to prevent fetal compromise.
- Appendicitis presents with abdominal pain, nausea, vomiting, fever and leucocytosis. Serial white cell counts may have to be done as pregnancy is usually associated with a mild leucocytosis. The position of the appendix changes with advancing gestation, hence the site of pain may be higher up on the right side than in non-pregnant women. A delay in treatment may mean risking perforation, peritonitis and sepsis with risks of preterm labour and fetal demise. Therefore, a laparotomy should not be delayed. A right paramedian incision over the area of maximum tenderness allows better access and a choice of extending the incision if needed. Postoperatively, one must carefully monitor for the onset of preterm labour.
- Another cause of abdominal pain can be due to intestinal obstruction mainly due to adhesions, volvulus, hernias or intussusception. There may be associated constipation, distension and high-pitched bowel sounds. An erect X-ray will reveal multiple air-fluid levels and dilated loops of bowel. If no signs of strangulation are present, conservative management in the

form of intravenous fluids and nasogastric suction should be tried. Early surgery after correcting fluid and electrolyte imbalance should be undertaken with a vertical midline incision. Adequate maternal oxygenation and uterine perfusion should be ensured during anaesthesia which may either be general or regional.

- Acute cholecystitis presents with sudden onset of right upper quadrant or epigastric colicky pain, nausea, fever and abdominal tenderness. Murphy's sign is less common in pregnancy. Ultrasound of the gallbladder and common bile duct will demonstrate gallstones in a majority of cases. Treatment includes conservative management in the first instance with analgesia, intravenous fluids, nasogastric suction and antibiotics. If these fail, or in case of suspicion of peritonitis, perforation or empyema of the gallbladder, a laparotomy will be necessary.
- Acute pyelonephritis occurs in 1–2% of pregnant women. Treatment is conservative in the form of intravenous fluids, analgesia and antibiotics.
- Acute pancreatitis, though rare in pregnancy (1 : 4000), carries a 10% mortality. The diagnostic test is raised serum amylase.

Q72. You are the on-call registrar when you are crash called to attend to a woman brought in to casualty after a major road traffic accident. She is unconscious, with shallow respiration, and is bleeding from multiple wounds. She is also 30 weeks pregnant. Justify your management.

A72.

- The principles of resuscitation of a pregnant patient are essentially the same as that of the non-pregnant woman with a few exceptions.
- An initial rapid primary survey should be performed, in which airway, breathing and circulation (ABC) are stabilized. The main priorities are airway with cervical spine stabilization. A patent airway is established using basic and advanced or surgical means. Chin lift or insertion of a nasopharyngeal airway may be required. Oral intubation will protect against aspiration.
- Supplementary oxygen must be administered. If a chest drain is required, it is inserted at a higher level than normal (3/4 intercostal space).
- It is important to treat fluid losses aggressively, as abnormalities in pulse, blood pressure and urine output may not become apparent until 20–30% of blood volume is lost because of the hypervolaemia of pregnancy. The fetus, however, will succumb much before this. Crystalloid infusions of up to 50% above that required in the non-gravid patient are often necessary to maintain the increased plasma volume.

- The pregnant trauma victim should be nursed at a 30 degree angle to the left to eliminate vena caval and aortic compression by the gravid uterus which will reduce venous return, cardiac output and uterine perfusion. The patient is best managed on a spinal board with a wedge, and if this is not available, manual displacement of the uterus should be done.
- A secondary survey is now conducted by the trauma team, which includes a head to toe examination of the victim, including a log roll and per rectal examination.
- Resuscitation of the mother is the treatment that best serves the fetus. Once the mother's condition is stabilized, the fetus should be evaluated by an ultrasonic Doppler probe to monitor the fetal heart rate.
- A cardiotocograph is then done and signs of compromise such as tachycardia, late decelerations, loss of baseline variability or bradycardia are noted. The uterus should be assessed for abruption or rupture. In case of fetal compromise, a caesarean delivery should be conduced as soon as the mother is stabilized.
- If aggressive cardiopulmonary resuscitation with a properly positioned patient is not successful after 5 min, caesarean delivery must be performed as soon as possible. This procedure will immediately relieve the vena caval compression and increase the chances of survival of both infant and mother. CPR must be continued throughout the procedure until spontaneous and effective cardiac activity occurs.
- It is important to be aware of the particular problems in resuscitating a pregnant woman, while being adept at the basic principles of resuscitation.

Q73. You are called urgently to see a woman who delivered a baby 2 h ago and subsequently complains of sudden chills, sweating, breathlessness followed by shock, cyanosis and cardiovascular collapse. Critically appraise your management.

A73.

- The above signs and symptoms may be consistent with a number of obstetric emergencies. The initial management however, will be the same and follow universal principles of resuscitation.
- The ABCs (airway, breathing and circulation) are stabilized. Endotracheal intubation and mechanical ventilation using inspired oxygen concentrations of 100% delivered by positive pressure and PEEP (positive end expiratory pressure) should be carried out. Placement of two wide bore intravenous cannulae to deliver large volumes of fluid and an intrarterial catheter to monitor blood pressure, arterial blood gases and a central

venous catheter to monitor cardiac status, pulmonary pressures and fluid balance should be done.

- The differential diagnosis in this case will include pulmonary thromboembolism, amniotic fluid embolism, a toxic reaction to a local anaesthetic, haemorrhagic shock or a cerebrovascular accident. Investigations which will help in reaching a diagnosis include chest X-ray, ventilation perfusion lung scan and estimation of blood coagulation factors which will become abnormal in DIC secondary to amniotic fluid embolism. A definitive diagnosis of amniotic fluid embolism can only be made by postmortem examination. A cerebrovascular embolism is distinct from amniotic fluid embolism by the absence of cyanosis, hypotension and pulmonary oedema. Haemorrahgic shock is ruled out by careful examination to exclude bleeding, the absence of central cyanosis and CVP.

  TPA

- There is no clear regime of drug therapy to reverse the symptoms of amniotic fluid embolism. Drug therapy and other treatment are supportive to improve the ventilation/perfusion ratio, maintenance of adequate blood pressure and treatment of DIC. Drugs that may play a role include salbutamol, dopamine, aminophylline and hydrocortisone.
- If a pulmonary embolism is strongly suspected, anticoagulation should be started immediately and ventilation perfusion scan carried out.
- Bleeding secondary to DIC requires blood replacement using fresh whole blood, or if unavailable, packed red cell and frozen plasma. Cryoprecipitate and platelet transfusion are also required.
- Uterine bleeding should be controlled by massage and use of intravenous oxytocin. If bleeding is unresponsive, one should consider an examination under anaesthetic and exploration for retained placenta or membranes or a search for cervical or uterine lacerations.

Q74. A woman has her first eclamptic fit immediately after delivery in hospital. What principles underlie her subsequent management?
A74.
- The immediate management is to secure the airway and position the patient appropriately.
- Urgent senior obstetric and anaesthetic help should be requested.
- The labour ward should have an agreed protocol which should be followed.
- Further fits must be prevented. The drug of choice is magnesium sulphate.
- The blood pressure must be controlled to prevent CVA and hypertensive cardiac failure by the use of rapidly acting drugs.

- Oliguria may complicate renal damage and fluid overload may precipitate pulmonary oedema. The volume of crystalloid should be tightly controlled.
- Monitoring includes:
  pulse oximetry
  tendon reflexes, respiratory rate
  blood pressure
  urine output
  biochemical and haematological indices.
- The patient is best managed on a high dependency unit or intensive care under a single lead clinician.

Q75. A 32-year-old primiparous woman at 34 weeks gestation is admitted with a blood pressure of 140/90 mmHg and 2+ proteinuria. She starts complaining of severe epigastric pain, nausea and vomiting. Serum biochemical values are as follows: aspartate transaminase 100 μmol/L, urates 600 μmol/L, plasma glucose 1.4 mmol/L, platelets 75 × 10^9/L. Critically appraise how you will reach a diagnosis and manage the case.
A75.

- The most likely diagnosis in this case is acute fatty liver of pregnancy, the differential diagnosis being HELLP syndrome. It is distinguished from the latter by mild hypertension and proteinuria, profound hypoglycaemia and marked hyperuricaemia.
- A liver biopsy though diagnostic, is seldom undertaken because of the possibility of associated coagulopathy. MRI, CT scanning and ultrasound scanning can be used as alternative methods of diagnosis, with signs of fatty infiltration of the liver being looked for.
- A multidisciplinary team consisting of a senior obstetrician, liver specialists and neonatologists should be involved in the care of the woman in an intensive care setting.
- Complications may include fulminant hepatic failure, disseminated intravascular coagulation and renal failure.
- Optimal management involves immediate treatment of coagulopathy, hypertension and hypoglycaemia followed by delivery. Plasmapharesis, ventilation and dialysis may be required in certain cases.
- In case of fulminant hepatic failure, a liver transplant may be required.

Q76. You are asked to see a woman suffering from puerperial pyrexia. Outline your management.

A76.

- Puerperial pyrexia is defined as a temperature elevation of 38°C on two occasions after the first 24 h following delivery. Familiarizing oneself with the antenatal, intrapartum and postnatal course will enable one to make a *Prolonged differential diagnosis of the underlying cause and help in commencing treatment.*

- The differential diagnosis of puerperial pyrexia includes endometritis, deep vein thrombosis, abscesses, haematomas, septic pelvic vein thrombophlebitis, infections of abdominal or perineal wounds, urinary tract infections, chest infections, mastitis and breast abscesses.

- A history of prolonged rupture of membranes, chorioamnionitis, colonization with β-haemolytic *Streptococcus*, *Chlamydia* and *Gardnerella*, repeated vaginal examinations and the use of internal fetal monitoring should be obtained.

- Pyrexia associated with uterine tenderness and a foul vaginal discharge points towards uterine infections. Genital cultures may not be helpful as the flora in normal women resembles that of women with endometritis. Broad-spectrum antibiotics in the form of gentamycin and clindamycin should be used in women without renal complications.

- In case of retained products with endometritis, evacuation should be carried out after 24 h of intravenous antibiotic therapy.

- Pyrexia along with signs of calf tenderness or pulmonary symptoms should alert one to the possibility of a deep vein thrombosis. Doppler ultrasonography may confirm the diagnosis. A ventilation/perfusion scan should be ordered in case of chest symptoms and treatment started immediately with therapeutic doses of heparin.

- Careful examination for the presence of a vulval haematoma should be carried out, including a rectovaginal examination. Small haematoma may be treated with cold compresses but larger ones should undergo surgical evacuation with suction drainage and broad-spectrum antibiotics.

- Contamination by catheters, urinary retention and asymptomatic bacteriuria of pregnancy may contribute to cystitis or pyelonephritis, with symptoms of frequency, dysuria, hesitancy, urgency, incontinence, flank pain, nausea and chills. A mid-stream sample of urine should be taken for culture and sensitivity, and treatment with antibiotics started in case of positive microscopy.

- Fever along with breast pain and erythema suggests a diagnosis of mastitis. In case of a fluctuant mass, ultrasonography should be carried out to rule out a breast abscess. Expressing of milk and a penicillinase-resistant β-lactam such as dicloxacillin (erythromycin if allergic to penicillin) should be started. In case of an abscess, the pus should be drained, taking culture swabs at the same time and starting a prolonged course of antibiotics. Breastfeeding can continue with mastitis, though is generally stopped in case of breast abscesses.

Q77. A midwife calls you urgently to a normal delivery, which has just occurred. The baby is pale and gasping. You know the paediatrician is currently in theatre attending a section. Describe your actions clearly.
A77.

- The key steps in any resuscitation are airway, breathing and circulation (ABC).
- This baby has not established satisfactory spontaneous respiration so is likely to require immediate resuscitation, at least at a basic level.
- You need suction, oxygen and a warm well-lit area to assess the baby. This is most easily found on a neonatal resuscitaire which should be obtained if not already in the room.
- Ensure cord is clamped.
- Place baby on resuscitaire, offer facial oxygen by mask, and assess Apgar score rapidly (score 0–10, 0–2 each for respiration, heart rate, colour, reaction to stimulus and movement). If score is 3 or less, call for help immediately.
- AIRWAY: is airway clear? Inspect nose and mouth and ask about any history of blood or meconium at delivery. Clear nostrils with suction catheter.
- Enquire rapidly for history of:
  opiate administration in past 4 h
  any suspicion of fetal distress prior to delivery
  any delivery complication
  any known or suspected abnormality.
- Is baby dysmorphic or abnormal in appearance? All of the above should take less than 1 min.
- BREATHING: are the baby's gasps becoming more frequent and regular, with a heart rate (best assessed by feeling the base of the cord) of greater than 100 per minute? If so, continue to administer O_2 by mask and reassess.
- If the baby's HR is 60–100 or gasps remain erratic, the baby requires assisted respiration. Check airway is clear, apply correctly sized mask over baby's *nose and mouth*, and ventilate using bag or T-piece connector provided.
- Initial 'rescue' breaths of 1–2 s each ×5 (to inflate lungs) then continue ventilating at 30 b.p.m.
- If heart rate does not rapidly increase and colour improve, call again for help.

- CIRCULATION: if HR is less than 60, the baby requires circulatory assistance (external cardiac massage) as well as respiratory support as above. Two resuscitators are needed, one to ventilate, and the other to provide external cardiac massage at 120 per minute (use 1st and 2nd fingers to press over lower third of the baby's sternum aiming to depress it by about 1 cm each beat)
- When the baby has recovered or help has arrived take the opportunity to communicate to the parents what has happened.

Q78. You are called upon to urgently review a woman who had a normal delivery 40 min ago. Following this she started trickling blood vaginally. Initial measures taken by the midwife have not halted the bleeding. These included starting an oxytocin infusion intravenously and inspecting the perineum which appears to be intact. The placenta and membranes have also been inspected and appear complete. The woman continues to bleed and the estimated blood loss by now is around 900 mL. Critically appraise the steps you will take to manage this emergency.

A78.

- Urgent action needs to be taken to control the bleeding and replace the blood loss that has already occurred. Senior help in the form of the consultant obstetrician and anaesthetist must be summoned immediately, and the haematologist informed of the urgent need for blood products.
- Intravenous access with two large bore intravenous cannulae must be ensured, and if not already done, blood sent off urgently for cross-matching of at least 6 units of blood along with a coagulation screen.
- Fluid replacement with colloids or crystalloids should be done while waiting for the blood to be cross-matched. A central venous line may have to be inserted if the bleeding continues, to monitor fluid balance.
- The strength of the oxytocin infusion should be checked, with a minimum of 40 iu infused in 500 mL Hartmann's solution over 4 h.
- An examination under anaesthesia may be required if the woman continues to bleed to investigate the cause of the haemorrhage. The perineum should be rechecked to look for tears, and bimanual compression of the uterus carried out. In case of uterine atony, prostaglandin F_2 (carboprost) can be given intramuscularly or intramyometrially in a dose of 250 μg and repeated every 15 min up to 8 doses.
- Misoprostol, a prostaglandin E_1 analogue, can be given orally or rectally as an alternative uterotonic agent.
- Uterine packing with abdominal packs may be attempted. Alternatively, tamponade may be applied with the use of a Sengstaken–Blakemore tube

or a Foley catheter with a large balloon filled with 100 mL saline. This is later deflated slowly, when the blood loss and any clotting abnormalities have been corrected.

- Massive postpartum haemorrhage may lead to the onset of clotting abnormalities, and clotting factors will need to be replaced. A unit of fresh frozen plasma should be given for every 4 units of blood transfused, and a platelet infusion may be required if the platelet count falls below 50×10^9/dL. If bleeding continues, defective coagulation should be corrected before undertaking a laparotomy.
- Uterine artery ligation should be done bilaterally by a surgeon skilled in the technique. Alternatively, Internal artery ligation may be attempted. Embolization of the internal iliac and uterine vessels may be attempted by a radiologist skilled in this technique. The last resort, however, is a subtotal or total abdominal hysterectomy, though direct compression of uterine bleeding sites with a brace suture has also been tried with success.

Q79. 'Domestic violence often goes unnoticed and unreported.' Critically appraise how you will recognize signs of an abusive relationship and what steps you would take to help the victim of such abuse, with particular reference to the antenatal period.

A79.

- Health professionals are in a unique position whereby they come into close contact with victims of spousal abuse, and can intervene to stop it. In order to do this, they need to be trained in identifying, treating and referring victims of abuse.
- Domestic violence can be conceptualized as existing as a continuum from verbal or psychological abuse to severe physical abuse. Victims of such abuse may present with stress-related symptoms of victimization such as sleep disturbance, chronic abdominal or pelvic pain, frequent urinary or vaginal infections and dyspareunia, chronic headaches and frequent use of pain medication.
- A woman involved in abusive relationships may appear frightened, evasive, passive or jumpy. She may be reluctant to speak in the presence of her partner, who may answer her questions for her. Other symptoms may be repeated presentations with depression, or substance misuse and alcohol abuse.
- Common injuries to look out for in victims of domestic violence include contusions, fractures or sprains, injuries to head, neck, chest, breasts and abdomen, or multiple site injuries and injuries during pregnancy. The

victim's explanation of the mechanism of injury is usually inconsistent with the physical presentation or there may be a delay in seeking medical care.

- Pregnancy places a woman at increased risk of being abused, and because of the great risk to both mother and baby, assessment for abuse should be incorporated into prenatal and postpartum care. The partner may limit the victim's access to antenatal care, resulting in missed or cancelled appointments. When she does turn up for appointments, the spouse may insist on accompanying her. It is important to devise ways and means of interviewing the woman alone and encouraging her to own up to the abuse. Simple, direct questions about abuse should be incorporated into routine examinations. If she desires, information should be offered on legal and social services, and the telephone numbers for local and national helplines left in the waiting rooms or toilets.

Chapter 4
Maternal and fetal infections

Chapter 4: **Questions**

Answers are on pp. 99–105

Q80. A general practitioner rings you worried about a patient of his who has developed chicken pox. She is 18 weeks pregnant. What advice would you give?

Q81. A woman is diagnosed to be HIV positive at 12 weeks of pregnancy. Critically appraise the management of the rest of her pregnancy.

Q82. A woman presents at 36 weeks gestation with herpetic lesions on her vulva. There is no history of genital herpes simplex in the past. Justify your management of the pregnancy.

Q83. A woman presents to the labour ward in threatened preterm labour with intact membranes. She is 29 weeks pregnant. A high vaginal swab taken at the time reveals a heavy growth of β-haemolytic *Streptococcus*. Justify your management of the pregnancy.

Q84. Critically appraise the methods of reducing vertical transmission of HIV in pregnant women.

Q85. A woman suspected of being a chronic hepatitis B carrier books in to your antenatal clinic. Justify your approach to her management.

Q86. A TORCH screen done on a pregnant woman in the second trimester reveals high titres of IgG and IgM to *Toxoplasma* infection. Justify your management.

Chapter 4: **Answers**

Q80. A general practitioner rings you worried about a patient of his who has developed chicken pox. She is 18 weeks pregnant. What advice would you give?

A80.

- Primary varicella zoster infection is caused by a DNA virus which is transmitted by respiratory droplets and close personal contact. There may be fever, malaise and a pruritic maculopapular rash, which become vesicles and crust over.
- The diagnosis of primary varicella infection should be confirmed by detecting IgM antibodies in the patient's serum.
- The pregnant woman with varicella should be isolated from all other pregnant women and neonates.
- Primary infection is more severe in adults and pneumonia can occur in up to 10% of cases. It is imperative to be vigilant for any chest symptoms and to admit into hospital under the respiratory physicians if this happens.
- In case of severe disease intravenous aciclovir should be considered if the woman has been seen within 24 h of developing the rash. This may reduce severity and duration of the illness.
- In this case, as the chicken pox has developed at less than 20 weeks, there is a 2% risk of developing the congenital varicella syndrome in the fetus. This includes skin scarring, eye defects in the form of cataracts, microphthalmia or chorioretinitis; hypoplasia of the limbs and neurological abnormalities. The patient should be thoroughly counselled about this risk and a detailed mid-trimester scan carried out at around 20 weeks to look for any abnormalities.
- Neonatal ophthalmic examination should be arranged at birth.

Q81. A woman is diagnosed to be HIV positive at 12 weeks of pregnancy. Critically appraise the management of the rest of her pregnancy.

A81.

- HIV type 1 has become the scourge of the modern world with over 1% of the world's sexually active population being affected with the virus which is the main cause of the AIDS pandemic. There is a great advantage in detecting the virus early on in pregnancy as active measures can be taken to reduce viral load and prevent vertical transmission.
- A detailed history and examination should be undertaken including possible modes of transmission. Screening for other sexually transmitted diseases should be undertaken. A history of intravenous drug abuse

should be elicited with appropriate investigations and referral if still ongoing. Baseline serology for cytomegalovirus and toxoplasmosis should also be undertaken.

- In case of a positive history of intravenous drug abuse a full hepatitis screen including hepatitis B and C should be carried out.
- Management of the woman should be undertaken in conjunction with an HIV expert.
- Screening for viral load should be undertaken. This will facilitate decisions regarding appropriate antiretroviral treatment. This is done by estimating CD4 counts in the serum and comparing CD4 and CD8 ratios. They should also be tested in each trimester, with a drop below $200/mm^3$ requiring antimicrobial prophylaxis for *Pneumocystis carinii* along with combination antiretroviral therapy.
- Highly active antiretroviral therapy (HAART) is now available and has been successful in reducing plasma viraemia to undetectable levels in over 50% of patients. The decision on combination therapy will depend upon viral load and clinical condition, with a combination of protease inhibitors and nucleoside analogue reverse transcriptase inhibitors being favoured in case of a high viral load.
- Monotherapy with zidovudine in the third trimester is appropriate for women who are clinically well with a low viral load, as transmission of the virus mainly occurs around delivery. Treatment with one drug minimizes side-effects and as it is given for a short duration of time, the development of resistance too is minimized. There is a reduction in frequency of transmission by an average of 68%.
- Elective caesarean sections reduce the risk of vertical transmission significantly, with a combination of prophylactic zidovudine and caesarean section reducing transmission to 2%. This is protective only however, if caesarean section is performed before labour or soon after rupture of membranes.
- Breastfeeding doubles the rate of transmission of the virus and should be discouraged.
- Birthweight may be slightly reduced and thus serial scanning should be undertaken to monitor fetal condition and growth.
- Emphasis should be placed on education and counselling of the patient and her partner. Contact tracing and contraceptive advice forms an important part of this.

Q82. A woman presents at 36 weeks gestation with herpetic lesions on her vulva. There is no history of genital herpes simplex in the past. Justify your management of the pregnancy.

A82.

- Neonatal herpes viral infection is a severe systemic illness with a high perinatal morbidity rate. There is a strong association with vertical transmission from affected mothers and various measures can be undertaken to prevent this from occurring.

- Evidence of infection must first be confirmed. This is done by type-specific serology and viral cultures from genital lesions. Primary and secondary herpes infection is differentiated by detecting the presence of HSV-2 antibodies. Their absence would indicate a primary infection.

- The woman should be treated with acyclovir which not only reduces the duration and severity of symptoms but is also associated with reducing the duration of viral shedding. Daily suppressive acyclovir used in the last 4 weeks of pregnancy has been shown to reduce vertical transmission of the virus. There is no evidence of harmful effects on the fetus.

- The woman should be referred to a genitourinary specialist to advise on management and screen for other sexually transmitted infections.

- As the primary infection has occurred in the third trimester, it is recommended that an elective caesarean section should be considered at term. This is because transmission mainly occurs via contact of the fetus with infected maternal fluids and lesions during passage through the birth canal, which is prevented by caesarean section.

- If the woman opts for a vaginal delivery, intravenous acyclovir during labour will minimize viral shedding and should be given to the mother. The neonate should also be administered intravenous acyclovir at birth.

- In the case of a vaginal delivery, invasive procedures such as fetal scalp electrode monitoring, fetal blood sampling, and instrumental deliveries should be avoided to minimize the risk of transmission.

- In case serology testing reveals that the episode is a recurrence, there is very little risk of transmission to the fetus and the mother should be reassured. In this case a vaginal delivery should be allowed unless there are obstetric indications for a caesarean section. The practice of repeated viral cultures to detect recurrence close to term is not recommended.

Q83. A woman presents to the labour ward in threatened preterm labour with intact membranes. She is 29 weeks pregnant. A high vaginal swab taken at the time reveals a heavy growth of β-haemolytic *Streptococcus*. Justify your management of the pregnancy.

A83.

- Group B *Streptococcus* has become recognized as one of the most important causes of neonatal infection and must be taken seriously. Threatened preterm labour may end with a preterm delivery in 5–10% of cases and should be appropriately managed.

- A woman who presents at 29 weeks gestation with premature contractions should be thoroughly screened for infections including a temperature check and white cell count along with a high vaginal swab, a mid-stream specimen of urine for culture and C reactive protein estimation.
- Careful appraisal of the maternal and fetal condition should be undertaken including ultrasonography to ascertain fetal growth, morphology and presentation and measurement of amniotic fluid volume.
- A cervical assessment should be carried out to determine if actual preterm labour is occurring. This is also useful in serving as a reference point for when actual labour supervenes.
- As long as intrauterine infection has been ruled out, steroids to promote fetal lung maturity in the event of a preterm delivery should be administered.
- Tocolysis with β-sympathomimetic drugs should be considered for at least 48 h while the steroids take effect. They have not been shown to have a benefit beyond this period of time.
- Neonatal mortality with group B *Streptococcus* is estimated to be around 5%. It is a leading cause of neonatal septicaemia and meningitis in the first 2 months of life. Though 6–30% of women in the general population will be colonized with GBS, antepartum treatment with antibiotics has not shown to be of benefit with the current recommendations being intrapartum chemoprophylaxis. In this case however, because of the additional risk factor of preterm labour, treatment should be started with intravenous penicillin G. Alternative drugs include ampicillin, clindamycin or erythromycin in penicillin-sensitive patients.
- It is very important to counsel the patient and her partner about the mode of delivery in case labour supervenes and the possible prognosis for the baby in view of its prematurity. This should be done in conjunction with a neonatologist. Adequate facilities for neonatal care at that particular gestation should be available and if not, transfer to a tertiary centre with these facilities should be done.

Q84. Critically appraise the methods of reducing vertical transmission of HIV in pregnant women.

A84.

- Vertical transmission of HIV is around 14% in the west and up to 40% in the developing world. There are several measures that can be taken to limit the number affected.
- Transmission to the fetus mainly depends upon viral load. This can be reduced by warning against unprotected intercourse while pregnant. Women with sexually transmitted diseases should be counselled about testing for HIV as they are at a higher risk of contracting the virus. Antenatal HIV testing should be made universal and easily available. Termination of a pregnancy may be discussed in context.
- Highly active antiretroviral drug therapy (HAART) should be recommended for all women with a high viral load. Monotherapy with zidovudine in the third trimester when used in women who are clinically well with a low viral load, reduces transmission by up to 68%. This is because transmission of the virus mainly occurs around the time of delivery.
- Elective caesarean sections, when undertaken before the onset of labour and spontaneous rupture of membranes, along with prophylactic zidovudine can reduce vertical transmission to up to 2%.
- Invasive procedures such as cordocentesis, amniocentesis, fetal blood sampling and the use of fetal scalp electrodes should be avoided.
- In case a vaginal delivery is unavoidable, episiotomy should be avoided and the forceps used to deliver the baby rather than a vacuum extractor, if an instrumental delivery is required.
- Breastfeeding should be discouraged, as the risk of vertical transmission increases by up to 14%.

Q85. A woman suspected of being a chronic hepatitis B carrier books in to your antenatal clinic. Justify your approach to her management.

A85.

- Of women with the hepatitis B virus 10% go on to become chronic carriers. They are recognized by the presence of hepatitis B S antigen (HBsAg) in the serum. These women may develop chronic active hepatitis, chronic persistent hepatitis and, rarely, fulminant infection. Vertical transmission may occur, usually at delivery, in around 1% of cases. Late sequelae of chronic HBs virus carriage include hepatic cirrhosis and primary hepatocellular carcinoma, more common in infants of carrier mothers who fail to respond to immunization at birth.

- Confirmation of carrier status is carried out by screening for HBsAg in the serum. Acute infection can be ruled out by carrying out a full hepatitis B viral screen which includes hepatitis B e antigen (HBeAg), antibody to HBsAg (anti-HBs) and antibody to hepatitis B core antigen (anti-HBc).
- The woman should be reassured that there are no teratogenic effects of chronic carriage of the virus and no adverse pregnancy events.
- Serological studies for hepatitis C and HIV infection should be carried out, with prior counselling.
- Infection control measures should be taken with all body products, and medical staff warned of biohazards due to chronic carriage.
- The newborn should undergo active and passive immunoprophylaxis. Hepatitis B immunoglobulin (HBIg) should be administered within 12 h of birth, followed by three doses of the hepatitis B vaccine. The initial dose is given within 7 days of birth, followed by doses at 1 and 6 months. HBsAg is tested at 12–15 months.
- Family members of the woman should be counselled regarding the risk of transmission, and tested if appropriate.

Q86. A TORCH screen done on a pregnant woman in the second trimester reveals high titres of IgG and IgM to *Toxoplasma* infection. Justify your management.
A86.
- Primary maternal infection with toxoplasmosis in the third trimester can result in fetal infection in up to 65% of cases. However, the later the infection, the less severe the damage.
- Acute infection is confirmed by a fourfold increase in IgG titres in blood samples taken 3 weeks apart, by the ELISA test. Alternatively, high IgM titres also indicate acute infection.
- Toxoplasmosis in the fetus manifests as a syndrome of chorioretinitis, micro- or hydrocephaly, intracerebral calcifications and mental retardation.
- Diagnosis of fetal infection is made by a PCR test on amniotic fluid obtained by amniocentesis. The risks of this procedure, including the 1% risk of miscarriage, should be discussed with the mother before undertaking it. Additional tests include ultrasonography which may reveal cerebral calcifications, or cordocentesis for collection of fetal blood and diagnostic testing.
- Spiramycin (3 g/day), should be administered to the mother in order to prevent fetal infection as soon as the diagnosis is made.

- If fetal infection is proven by amniotic fluid or fetal blood testing, the option of termination of the pregnancy should be discussed with the parents in view of the potentially severe consequences of fetal infection.
- Intrauterine antibiotic treatment with spiramycin for maternal infection coupled with pyramethamine and sulphonamides for documented fetal infection can be tried.

Chapter 5
Neonatology

Chapter 5: **Questions**

Answers are on pp. 108–113

Q87. At a postnatal visit after an uneventful pregnancy and delivery, the mother asks you if her baby's persisting jaundice is significant or worrying. Baby is 4 weeks old and visibly yellow. What salient questions would you ask and what investigations, if any, are needed?

Q88. You are asked to see a baby on the delivery ward because the baby's sex is not definite. What are you going to do? What may the problem be?

Q89. You have successfully delivered a baby with minor shoulder dystocia. When you visit mother and baby a few hours later, the mother is very agitated and angry and tells you that baby is not moving his right arm normally. Explain your management of this case.

Q90. What, if any, are the advantages to the baby of being breast fed in the early weeks of life?

Q91. Antenatal steroids are recommended by the RCOG for any woman who is expected to deliver prematurely. What are the advantages and disadvantages for the baby of this policy?

Q92. Due to poor placental function and poor fetal growth, your senior colleague has recommended caesarean section at 30 weeks to your patient. As you admit her she asks you what is likely to happen to the baby. What will you discuss with her?

Q93. Your pregnant patient is an ex-heroin addict who is now on a methadone programme. What complications may be anticipated for her baby at birth and afterwards?

Chapter 5: **Answers**

Q87. At a postnatal visit after an uneventful pregnancy and delivery, the mother asks you if her baby's persisting jaundice is significant or worrying. Baby is 4 weeks' old and visibly yellow. What salient questions would you ask and what investigations if any are needed?

A87.

- Persisting jaundice after 14 days is abnormal and cannot be assumed to be 'physiological'. Further enquiry and investigation are always needed.
- Is there a family history of haemolytic conditions such as G6PD deficiency (commoner in those of Mediterranean extraction) or spherocytosis (an autosomal dominant condition commonly leading to splenectomy in adult life)? An affected baby may have been jaundiced since day 1 and may have become anaemic. G6PD assay and FBC/film will be needed.
- Is there any evidence of any abnormal antibodies in mother's bloods checked antenatally leading to blood group incompatibility between mother and baby, presenting as above. If mother is group O and father is group A or B there may be ABO incompatibility. Group and direct antiglobulin test on baby's blood will be needed.
- Was there an illness in pregnancy, which may have put baby at risk for a congenital viral infection?
- Is baby thriving, asymptomatic, breast-fed, with clear urine and brown/yellow stools? If so this is likely to be 'breast milk' jaundice. Blood for total/direct reacting bilirubin will exclude liver disease if the direct reacting fraction is near zero or zero.
- All babies are offered a screening blood test at 6–10 days which screens for elevated TSH, so congenital hypothyroidism should already have been excluded in this baby.
- If baby is at all unwell or not thriving or has dark urine or pale stools, urgent paediatric referral is needed to exclude underlying infective, metabolic or structural liver disease. Biliary atresia presents with prolonged jaundice, the direct reacting fraction of bilirubin will be elevated, and liver enzymes will also be abnormally raised. This is an urgent diagnosis to make as treatment success varies inversely with age at diagnosis.

Q88. You are asked to see a baby on the delivery ward because the baby's sex is not definite. What are you going to do? What may the problem be?

A88.

- This not uncommon problem must be dealt with sensitively.
- Risks are:

that the family reject the baby

that the baby is reared as the 'wrong' sex

that the baby has a potentially serious medical condition, such as viriliza-
tion related to congenital adrenal hyperplasia (CAH), a metabolic defect
leading to deficient production of cortisol, and is in danger of a salt-
losing crisis in the neonatal period.

- In the UK, the parents have 42 days before the baby's birth must be
registered. They should be informed of the uncertainty, and an explanation given that baby should not be named or registered until the 'correct'
sex can be determined.
- Initial investigations will include a chromosomal karyotype, and a pelvic
US to ascertain the presence or absence of a uterus or gonads.
- Blood for 17-hydroxyprogesterone assay, taken _after_ the age of 72 h, will
exclude the commonest form of CAH, due to 21-hydroxylase deficiency.
urea and electrolytes in blood and urine should be monitored.
- Baby will come into one of three broad categories: Testicular feminu
  - Inadequately virilized genetic male. There is likely to be non-
    production of testosterone, or loss of end-organ responsiveness to
    dihydrotestosterone which can be partial or complete. An hCG
    stimulation test may help in deciding appropriate best sex of rearing.
  - Masculinized genetic female. CAH should be excluded, maternal inges-
    tion of androgens during pregnancy should be investigated.
  - True hermaphrodite, with both ovarian and testicular tissue present.
    Such babies will require specialist investigation and treatment. These
    children are usually raised as females.

Q89. You have successfully delivered a baby with minor shoulder dystocia. When you visit mother and baby a few hours later, the mother is very
agitated and angry and tells you that baby is not moving his right arm
normally. Explain your management of this case.
A89.

- The possibilities here are
  clavicular fracture
  humerus fracture
  injury to upper roots of the brachial plexus leading to nerve dysfunction
  which may be temporary or permanent.
- Take mother's concerns seriously, listen to her, and assure her that you
  will ensure a prompt paediatric opinion. Do not assume that the problem
  is transient or trivial. Brachial injury is a recognized complication of
  shoulder dystocia and may well have been obstetrically unavoidable.

- Clear description and documentation of the delivery details are important in such cases for clinical and medicolegal reasons.
- Baby will need a chest X-ray/arm X-ray after paediatric clinical examination, to exclude a fracture. This may also show any associated ipsilateral diaphragmatic weakness.
- The upper roots of the brachial plexus, originating from C3/4/5, are likely to be involved in any nerve injury. Typically, there is a loss of shoulder abduction, arm external rotation, and wrist extension. The 'Moro' response will be asymmetrical. The arm may assume an internally rotated posture (waiter's tip). This condition is called Erb's palsy.
- Management
  - Clavicle fracture; no specific treatment. Will heal spontaneously with formation of exuberant callus forming a lump which will resolve.
  - Humerus fracture with no nerve involvement: arm is usually strapped against the body for comfort for a few days. Should heal spontaneously with natural remodelling overcoming any minor fracture angulation.
  - Brachial plexus injury. If this does not resolve within 2–3 weeks, it may not resolve completely. Referral to an experienced plastic surgeon is indicated for the 10% of injuries in which this occurs.

Q90. What, if any, are the advantages to the baby of being breast fed in the early weeks of life?
A90.

- This method of feeding is best for babies and should be encouraged whenever possible.
- Bonding between mother and baby is promoted, enhancing baby's well-being.
- Epidemiologically, breast-fed babies have an overall lower infant mortality rate.
- Breast milk contains IgA, lysozyme, lymphocytes and macrophages, and transmits humoral and cellular immunity to the baby, particularly protecting baby's gut.
- *Lactobacillus* colonization of the gut is enhanced by the characteristics of human milk.
- Lactoferrin in human milk promotes lactobacilli and inhibits *E. coli* therefore reducing the risk of gastroenteritis.
- Electrolyte load is less than in formula milk thus reducing the risk of hypernatraemia in dehydration.
- Colostrum, produced in the first 2–3 days after birth, is rich in IgA and IgM promoting antiviral and antibacterial activity in the baby's gut.

- Formulae contains cow's milk protein, to which some individuals are allergic.
- If there is a strong FH of atopy, exclusive breastfeeding reduces the infant's incidence of eczema.
- Certain nutritional elements in breast milk such as taurine and very long chain fatty acids are important in neurodevelopment and *may* offer an advantage to breast-fed infants in aspects of later measured intelligence.
- Supply of milk is directed by the baby (by vigour and frequency of sucking) and therefore increase according to demand.
- Breast milk is warm and sterile and available 'on demand'.

Q91. Antenatal steroids are recommended by the RCOG for any woman who is expected to deliver prematurely. What are the advantages and disadvantages for the baby of this policy?

A91.

- Randomized controlled trials have demonstrated that single course administration of glucocorticoids in pregnancy improves postnatal lung function and reduces mortality in preterm babies without adverse consequences. This effect is seen even in the presence of ruptured membranes, extreme prematurity, or anticipated interval of less than 24 h before delivery. Treatment is effective if given within 7 days of delivery.
- Effects on the premature newborn include:
  - Increased tissue and alveolar surfactant, together with structural and biochemical lung maturation.
  - Possible maturation effects on brain and gastrointestinal tract.
  - Decreased mortality rate.
  - Decreased incidence and severity of RDS.
  - Decreased incidence of intraventricular haemorrhage.
  - Decreased incidence of significant patent ductus arteriosus.
  - Decreased length of stay on NNU.
- If preterm delivery does not occur within 7 days, repeated courses may be indicated but data is awaited as to the safety and efficacy of this.
- Caution is required because animal studies suggest that prenatal exposure to glucocorticoids restricts fetal growth, although this has not been found in human randomized controlled trials. In preterm babies, postnatal exposure to dexamethasone is associated with an increased risk of cerebral palsy. In experiments on immature neonatal animals, dexamethasone interferes with cerebral white matter development. Betamethasone has a lesser effect.

Q92. Due to poor placental function and poor fetal growth, your senior colleague has recommended caesarean section at 30 weeks to your patient. As you admit her she asks you what is likely to happen to the baby. What will you discuss with her?

A92.

- Babies with normal anatomy born in good condition at 30 weeks are very likely to survive, if cared for in a centre with modern neonatal facilities, survival is likely to be over 95%.
- There is the opportunity for this patient to receive a course of betamethasone at least 24 h prior to baby's delivery thus reducing the risk of respiratory distress syndrome, which at this gestation is about 50%.
- Baby may require stabilization at delivery by a paediatrician who will be present, and this may include intubation and ventilation if there is respiratory distress. Baby may require endotracheal surfactant, which is given shortly after birth. Ventilation, when needed, may be required for several days.
- He will require incubator care initially to maintain body temperature and may become jaundiced which will require phototherapy.
- Baby will require to be tube fed once able to tolerate enteral feeds and mother may wish to express breast milk for him, otherwise he will receive a formula milk modified for preterm babies. He is likely to start sucking feeds in about 4–5 weeks and to go home after 6–10 weeks.
- Mother may have the opportunity to care for her baby as soon as he is stable, participating in tube feeding, bathing and changing.
- Baby is at risk from complications such as acquired infection (pulmonary or general), persistent patent ductus arteriosus, or necrotizing enterocolitis. He is unlikely at this maturity to have an intraventricular haemorrhage, but is at risk for periventricular leucomalacia (which may be prenatal in origin) particularly as he is growth restricted.
- Long term he is at risk of neurodevelopmental delay, the risk increasing with reduced relative birth weight, and including the risks of cerebral palsy and of deafness, which is much commoner in ex-preterm babies.

Q93. Your pregnant patient is an ex-heroin addict who is now on a methadone programme. What complications may be anticipated for her baby at birth and afterwards?

A93.

- After birth the baby may be vulnerable to neonatal abstinence syndrome, a collection of symptoms which may not commence for 4–7 days after birth and may continue for several weeks. This affects feeding, sleeping, temperature control and behaviour.

- Characteristics are irritability, hypertonia, jitteriness, seizures, sneezing, tachycardia, diarrhoea and feeding difficulties. Management is with controlled reducing opiate administration orally to the baby, usually necessitating prolonged admission.
- Intrauterine exposure to narcotics can produce intrauterine growth retardation, poor postnatal growth and abnormal later development as well as an increased incidence of sudden infant death syndrome.
- At delivery the baby must not be given naloxone as this could provoke an acute withdrawal reaction.
- The possibility exists that the mother is abusing or has abused other drugs which may affect the fetus, for instance cocaine, which is associated with abruption, stillbirth and neonatal cerebral haemorrhage.
- The mother is at risk by her previous lifestyle of other diseases which can be passed to the baby, such as HIV (in which case intrapartum retroviral treatment is indicated), hepatitis B (in which case neonatal immunization ± immunoglobulin at birth is indicated), or hepatitis C.
- The family may have a dysfunctional lifestyle, leading to erratic child care and putting the child at risk after discharge, as well as increasing the likelihood of non-attendance or follow-up and difficulties with supervision. Social services should be made aware of the pregnancy and delivery.

Section B:
Gynaecology

Chapter 6
Reproductive medicine

Chapter 6: **Questions**

Answers are on pp. 119–125

Q94. Every couple should be offered full investigations for infertility after 1 year of failing to achieve a pregnancy. Critically discuss this statement.

Q95. A 25-year-old woman presents with excessive facial hair growth. Justify your management.

Q96. Discuss the aetiology and management of azoospermia.

Q97. A 32-year-old woman with primary infertility due to polycystic ovarian syndrome undergoes IVF treatment. A few days after embryo transfer, she is admitted as an emergency to the hospital with nausea and vomiting, severe abdominal pain and shortness of breath. A tense ascites is immediately recognizable. How will you go about managing this case?

Q98. Critically appraise the investigations for ascertaining tubal patency in the female.

Q99. A patient who has had infertility treatment discovers at the 6 weeks scan that she is expecting quadruplets. Justify your management and counselling.

Q100. Critically appraise the patient-related factors that influence the success of *in vitro* fertilization treatment.

Q101. A woman books at 8 weeks gestation in the antenatal clinic with a history of hyperprolactinaemia due to a macroprolactinoma. She is currently on cabergoline treatment. Critically appraise your management in view of her condition.

Q102. A woman presents to the assisted conception unit wishing to act as a surrogate mother for an infertile couple who have been unsuccessful in conceiving with IVF treatment. Critically appraise the advice you will offer to both parties.

Chapter 6: **Answers**

Q94. Every couple should be offered full investigations for infertility after 1 year of failing to achieve a pregnancy. Critically discuss this statement.
A94.

- 90% of couples will achieve a pregnancy after 1 year of trying, while 95% will do so after 2 years.
- In some cases, there are markers in the history to indicate the likelihood of a cause (e.g. pelvic inflammatory disease, irregular periods).
- The woman's age has a major impact on her chances of getting pregnant.
- The couple should be seen—if only for reassurance—whenever they express anxiety about their fertility, regardless of the duration.
- Investigations should be arranged taking into consideration the woman's age, any history markers, and the duration of infertility.
- At 1 year it is reasonable to investigate or (given a woman <35 years with no markers) to wait for another year, as 50% of those not pregnant by 1 year will become pregnant by 2 years.

Q95. A 25-year-old woman presents with excessive facial hair growth. Justify your management.
A95.

- Management will depend on history, examination and investigations.
- The aims of the management are to exclude a cause that may be dangerous (e.g. tumour); find a cause that may be treated accordingly; and offer medical, cosmetic and psychological support to the patient.
- Investigations should include hormonal profile (FSH, LH, testosterone, prolactin, TSH), and pelvic USS in all, and 17-OH progesterone in whom CAH is suspected.
- Specific causes are treated accordingly.
- In PCO or idiopathic causes the treatment will be either suppression of testosterone (combined oral contraceptive, cyproterone acetate) or suppression of 5-α reductase (finasteride).
- It takes up to 6 months to prevent new hair from growing, but the hair that had already grown will need electrolysis to be removed.

Q96. Discuss the aetiology and management of azoospermia.
A96.

- Azoospermia is the total absence of sperm from the ejaculate, which is a laboratory finding and not a diagnosis.

- It is present in 10–20% of infertile men.
- Two samples should be analysed, with proper instructions given on the method of collection. Centrifugation of the apparently azoospermic sample may yield sperm in 20% of cases. This is termed cryptozoospermia.
- *Pretesticular* azoospermia is due to lack of gonadotrophic stimulation of the testes, which could be congenital or acquired. Clinically there is hypogonadism, investigations include pituitary imaging, and treatment is with gonadotrophins if fertility is desired and with testosterone when fertility is not desired.
- *Testicular* azoospermia is due to testicular dysfunction/failure. It could be associated with karyotypic abnormalities or Y chromosome deletion (need genetic testing). Treatment is with attempted testicular sperm extraction (50% success) and ICSI.
- *Post-testicular* azoospermia is due to either obstruction (congenital bilateral absence of the vas—70% associated with CF carrier; infection; vasectomy) or retrograde ejaculation (postoperative; diabetic neuropathy). Treatment is either surgical correction of the obstruction or sperm retrieval and ICSI.

Q97. A 32-year-old woman with primary infertility due to polycystic ovarian syndrome undergoes IVF treatment. A few days after embryo transfer, she is admitted as an emergency to the hospital with nausea and vomiting, severe abdominal pain and shortness of breath. A tense ascites is immediately recognizable. How will you go about managing this case?
A97.
- The diagnosis is Ovarian Hyperstimulation Syndrome (OHSS). It is important to assess the severity of the patient's condition. Blood investigations include a full blood count including haematocrit, urea and electrolytes, renal and liver function tests and albumin along with a clotting screen. An ultrasound scan of the abdomen and pelvis is done to look for ovarian enlargement and degree of ascites. A chest ultrasound scan or X-ray is carried out to look for pleural effusions.
- Management of this condition is supportive, while waiting for it to resolve itself. Following admission, early correction of hypovolaemia is essential to improve renal function and reverse the haemoconcentration. Hartmann's solution or normal saline with added potassium if needed as the first line of therapy. Artificial plasma expanders such as Haemaccel can be used but will give temporary relief.
- There is a risk of thromboembolic complications and therefore prophylactic heparin is recommended. TED stockings should also be used.

- Urinary output and fluid balance should be closely monitored, together with blood pressure, temperature and respiratory rate. Daily abdominal girth measurement is a simple way of detecting deteriorating ascites. Haematological and biochemical parameters are indicators of disease progression and help in the management of fluid balance. They should initially be done daily. In case of poor urine output, catheterization may be needed.

- Abdominal paracentesis may be needed depending on the degree and progression of abdominal distension and the effect this has on respiratory effort. It should be done under ultrasound guidance to avoid damage to the large ovaries.

- A majority of cases will resolve spontaneously with supportive management. A laparotomy should be avoided except in those rare cases where torsion is suspected or there is evidence of significant intraperitoneal bleeding.

Q98. Critically appraise the investigations for ascertaining tubal patency in the female.

A98.

- Tubal patency testing is one of the initial investigations of female infertility. There are various tests that can be done, each with its pros and cons, depending upon the individual situation.

- Hysterosalpingography can be used as a screening test in low risk couples. There is a risk of infection of up to 1% in the general population and 3% in a high risk population. It should not be carried out in those with a recent history of pelvic inflammatory disease. Its advantages are the safety of usage and the delineation of the uterine cavity and fallopian tubes. Its disadvantage is the inability to assess the pelvic peritoneum.

- Diagnostic laparoscopy is an invasive procedure requiring a general anaesthetic with risks of visceral injury to the patient. However, careful inspection of all the pelvic organs and peritoneal folds is possible along with hydrotubation to test tubal patency. If used along with hysteroscopy, assessment of the uterine cavity can be done at the same time.

- Tubal patency can be assessed by ultrasound imaging with the help of a contrast medium or normal saline injected into the uterine cavity. It is non-invasive and safer than hysterosalpingography as irradiation is not used. Ovarian and uterine assessment can be carried out simultaneously. However, it is time consuming and requires trained personnel.

- Selective salpingography involves placing a small catheter directly into the proximal end of the fallopian tube and injecting a contrast agent. It overcomes tubal spasm, leading to less false positive results and improves the diagnosis of tubal disease. It may also be used therapeutically, by introducing a guide wire to break up intratubal adhesions. There is a risk of perforation approaching 5–10%.

- Falloscopy can be used to examine the entire length of the fallopian tubes but requires a great deal of expertise.
- There are a variety of methods by which tubal patency can be tested, and the one used will depend upon the individual patient, the setting of the hospital and its resources.

Q99. A patient who has had infertility treatment discovers at the 6 weeks scan that she is expecting quadruplets. Justify your management and counselling.

A99.

- Multiple pregnancies are a risk of modern drugs and superovulation regimes used in the treatment of infertility. Although perinatal mortality and morbidity have been dramatically reduced by advances in perinatal and neonatal care, the presence of higher order pregnancies is still associated with poor outcomes.
- There are mainly three options for the above couple. They either terminate the entire pregnancy, continue with the pregnancy with the inherent risk of miscarriage and morbidity, or they undergo multifetal pregnancy reduction or selective termination in order to maximize the chances of the pregnancy succeeding.
- Selective termination is mainly done by the ultrasound-guided transabdominal insertion of potassium chloride into the fetal heart. Other, less common methods are transvaginal aspiration of the embryos at about 6–7 weeks gestation and transcervical suction.
- In the case of quadruplets, the choice is of reduction to twins or a singleton pregnancy. As the greater number of fetuses are reduced, there is a higher risk of morbidity, therefore it is usually recommended to reduce the number to twins rather than a singleton.
- Most cases are performed between 9 and 12 weeks. Nuchal translucency should be measured on all the embryos prior to reduction. Monoamniotic twins have a greater risk of complications and should be reduced. Chorionic villus biopsy can be done before the procedure if genetic testing is required, followed by the reduction of any aneuploid fetuses. Alternatively, the pregnancy can be reduced to twins, and CVS performed afterwards.

↑ perinatal mostality/morbidity   Take home 60 –
↓ to twins – neurodeviptal delay   baby bar
                                                 – MFPR – 90 %.
Reproductive medicine   123

- There is an increasing risk of pregnancy loss and prematurity, hence these pregnancies should be closely monitored.

Q100. Critically appraise the patient-related factors that influence the success of *in vitro* fertilization treatment.

A100.

- There are key prognostic variables which determine the success of an IVF programme. They may be used to predict the likely outcome and chances of success for particular couples undergoing IVF treatment.
- Age of the female partner is an important determinant of success, the live birth rate being maximum for women undergoing IVF between 25 and 30 years, with a sharp decline in success rates beyond 35 years. A predicted live birth rate of 17% per cycle started at the age of 30 years declines to 7% and 2% at 40 and 45 years, respectively.
- Increasing duration of infertility is associated with a reduced success rate for IVF, after adjusting for age. After 10 years of infertility there is on average a live birth rate of 12% as compared to 15% for treatment after 3 years.
- The female indication of IVF does not seem to affect the chances of pregnancy.
- The presence of male factor will reduce the fertilization rate. This is overcome by using intracytoplasmic sperm injection.
- The presence of hydrosalpinx reduces the chances of success. Salpingectomy prior to IVF will increase the chances of success in such cases.
- Women with previous pregnancies have a higher live birth rate than those who have not been pregnant.
- The live birth rate is highest in the first cycle of IVF treatment and reduces in every successive cycle.

Q101. A woman books at 8 weeks gestation in the antenatal clinic with a history of hyperprolactinaemia due to a macroprolactinoma. She is currently on cabergoline treatment. Critically appraise your management in view of her condition.

A101.

- Pregnancy causes the pituitary to enlarge, and in this case it may cause the prolactinoma to enlarge with it. This in turn may give rise to clinical signs and symptoms, which is more likely in the event of a macroprolactinoma (15%).

- In the majority of cases of hyperprolactinaemia, there are no pregnancy complications. The woman should be reassured that there is no evidence of adverse obstetric outcome in the form of miscarriage or congenital anomalies.
- When pregnancy is confirmed, cabergoline should be discontinued.
- Serum prolactin levels are not helpful as they increase manifold in pregnancy.
- The patient should be instructed about possible symptoms of tumour expansion (headaches, visual disturbances). If these are reported, pituitary imaging (CT/MRI) should be performed. If confirmed, dopamine receptor agonists should be restarted.
- Dopamine receptor agonists are safe in pregnancy. They can also be used in breastfeeding, though the patient should be warned that they may suppress lactation.
- In cases refractory to medical treatment, surgery or radiotherapy may be needed, but are usually undertaken after delivery.

Q102. A woman presents to the assisted conception unit wishing to act as a surrogate mother for an infertile couple who have been unsuccessful in conceiving with IVF treatment. Critically appraise the advice you will offer to both parties.

A102.

- Surrogacy is an arrangement whereby a woman agrees to carry and give birth to a child on the understanding that it will be adopted by others at birth. The child may or may not be genetically related to the birth mother, with either her supplying the ovum with artificial insemination by the partner of the infertile couple, or with an embryo from the infertile couple.
- Commercial surrogacy is outlawed in the UK, and no money, apart from reasonable expenses for the birth mother during the pregnancy, should change hands.
- In UK law, the child of the surrogate mother remains hers and her husbands. Unless the child is adopted by the commissioning couple, they have no legal relationship with the child, or rights in law.
- A court order can be obtained soon after birth declaring that the child be treated for all purposes as though it were the child of the commissioning couple, if the application were made within 6 months of birth and the child has its home with the applicants. There should be a genetic relationship between the child and one of the parents, and all parties should give full and unconditional consent.

- The welfare of the child is of paramount importance, irrespective of the feelings of the other parties involved.
- Counselling should include the discussion of potential pregnancy complications, the possibility of fetal anomalies, and the short- and long-term relationship between the surrogate mother and the commissioning parents.

Chapter 7
Contraception

Chapter 7: Questions
Answers are on pp. 127–132

Q103. Male sterilization is safer and more effective than female sterilization. How will you justify this statement and counsel a couple who want to know about male sterilization?

Q104. A 48-year-old woman presents to your gynaecology clinic for advice regarding contraception. She has been on the combined oral contraceptive pill and wonders whether she should change it. Critically appraise the advice you would give her.

Q105. A 25-year-old woman attends your family planning clinic. She has never used the combined oral contraceptive pill and is considering starting it. She wants to know the benefits and risks involved. Critically appraise the advice you will impart to her.

Q106. A 22-year-old woman who has been on the combined oral contraceptive pill for the last 2 years presents to your family planning clinic saying she has missed three pills in succession. Justify the advice you will give her.

Q107. A 13-year-old girl comes to you requesting contraception. Her parents are not aware of the fact that she is sexually active. Critically appraise the way that you will approach the problem.

Q108. A woman comes to you wanting to know if the contraceptive implant would be suitable for her. She is a long-standing type I insulin-dependent diabetic, with no immediate plans to conceive. Critically appraise the advice you will give her.

Chapter 7: **Answers**

Q103. Male sterilization is safer and more effective than female sterilization. How will you justify this statement and counsel a couple who want
to know about male sterilization?
A103.

- Male sterilization, in the form of a vasectomy, is a procedure which
  involves division or removal of each vas with fascial interposition or
  diathermy.
- Male sterilization is performed under a local anaesthetic as compared to
  female sterilization, which usually requires a general anaesthetic. Thus it
  naturally cuts down on the inherent anaesthetic risks involved in the latter.
- Though both methods are associated with a failure rate, in the case of
  vasectomies, this is a $1:2000$ chance of pregnancy subsequent to the
  procedure as compared to female sterilization where the risk is $1:200$.
  Thus vasectomy is 10 times less likely to fail as compared to female
  sterilization. Pregnancies in both cases may occur many years following
  the procedure.
- Female sterilization is associated with a higher risk of ectopic pregnancies
  in case of failure, which is a definite life-threatening risk which can be
  avoided were the male to be sterilized instead. There are also the inherent
  risks of laparoscopy if this is the method adopted. These are mainly a risk
  of bowel and bladder or other visceral organ injury.
- Men who undergo a vasectomy should use alternative methods of contraception after the procedure until two consecutive semen analyses show
  azoospermia, 2–4 weeks apart, with the first test being at least 8 weeks
  after surgery.
- Men should be informed about the small risk of chronic testicular pain
  afterwards.

Q104. A 48-year-old woman presents to your gynaecology clinic for
advice regarding contraception. She has been on the combined oral
contraceptive pill and wonders whether she should change it. Critically
appraise the advice you would give her.
A104.

- Contraception in the perimenopausal age group needs to take into
  account the lowered fertility rate along with the increasing risk of cardiovascular disease.
- The woman can be advised that it is safe to continue with combined oral
  contraceptive until the age of 50 years provided she is a non-smoker with

no history of hypertension, obesity, family history of arterial disease or of breast cancer in young first degree relatives.

- She should be fully counselled about the association of the combined oral contraceptive and breast cancer, the risk of which increases in the peri-menopausal age group. There is one extra case of breast cancer in every 350 women on the combined pill.
- The other disadvantage is that they are prothrombotic and can mask the symptoms of the menopause. In cases of low endogenous oestrogen, vasomotor symptoms may appear on stopping the combined pill, along with a raised serum FSH and hormone replacement therapy can be offered with barrier methods of contraception for at least 12 months.
- If any of the contraindications listed above are present, the combined oral contraceptive should be discontinued, and an alternative method used.
- A rise in serum FSH levels is not a reliable method of diagnosing the onset of the menopause and thus discontinuing contraception because it fluc-tuates during the perimenopausal period. Repeatedly high levels along with other symptoms may point towards the onset of the menopause but even then it is recommended that some form of contraception such as barrier methods should be used for at least 12 months.

Q105. A 25-year-old woman attends your family planning clinic. She has never used the combined oral contraceptive pill and is considering starting it. She wants to know the benefits and risks involved. Critically appraise the advice you will impart to her.

A105.

- The combined oral contraceptive pill is a safe and reliable method of contraception. It has both risks and benefits associated with its use and the risks can be minimized by taking an accurate personal, medical and family history.
- The combined oral contraceptive pill offers extremely effective, non-intercourse related contraception. When used correctly, the pregnancy rate for the first year of use is less than 0.1%.
- The combined oral contraceptive pill causes a reduction in menstrual cycle disorders such as dysmenorrhoea, menorrhagia and premenstrual syndrome.
- It offers protection from benign breast disease and benign ovarian cysts. It also protects against pelvic inflammatory disease and ectopic pregnancies.
- Pill users are at a reduced risk of developing endometrial and ovarian cancer. After 1 year of use there is a reduction in endometrial cancer risk by 20% which increases to 50% after 4 years of use. Similarly, there is a

Menstl disorders
PID, ectopic
eudouetrical, Ovarian cancer
Rheumatoid arthritis, duod ulcers

VTE
MI
stroke
Breast cause

reduction in the risk of developing ovarian cancer by 40% after 3 years of use. In both these cancers, the reduction in risk persists for up to 15 years after stopping the pill, which is important because these cancers are mainly seen in postmenopausal women.

- As it causes less cyclical bleeding, there is a reduction in iron deficiency anaemia associated with menorrhagia. It may also cause a reduction in the size of fibroids and reduces the incidence of rheumatoid arthritis and duodenal ulcers, with symptomatic relief of endometriosis.
- There is an increased relative risk in the development of venous thromboembolism (VTE) in women taking the combined oral contraceptive pill, but the absolute risks are low and far outweighed by the benefits. The annual incidence of VTE in non-pill users is approximately 5 per 100 000 as compared to 15–30 per 100 000 in pill users. This is a small absolute risk when compared to the risk of VTE in pregnant women, which is 60 per 100 000 per year. The increased risk falls to that of non-users within 3 months of stopping the pill.
- There is an association between the use of the combined oral contraceptive pill and the occurrence of myocardial infarction. However, this is mainly related to smoking and other risk factors such as high blood pressure, diabetes and an abnormal lipid profile. Women who do not smoke and do not have other risk factors for cardiac disease are at little risk of myocardial infarction if they use the combined oral contraceptive pill.
- The combined oral contraceptive pill is associated with an increase in the risk of ischaemic and haemorrhagic stroke. In low risk women who are not hypertensive and who do not smoke, this risk is about 1.5 times that of non-users for ischaemic stroke but the risk of haemorrhagic stroke is no higher as compared to non-users. The risk of both types of stroke increases in women who are hypertensive and who smoke and this risk increases with age.
- There is an increase in the risk of breast cancer with pill use. This is a relative risk of 1.24 for current users and a progressively decreasing risk in the 10 years after stopping the pill. Again, the absolute risk is too small to change prescribing practices unless there is a strong genetic predisposition to breast cancer.

Q106. A 22-year-old woman who has been on the combined oral contraceptive pill for the last 2 years presents to your family planning clinic saying she has missed three pills in succession. Justify the advice you will give her.

A106.

- The contraceptive efficacy of the combined oral contraceptive pill is mainly dependent on the inhibition of ovulation. A minimum of seven consecutive pills are needed to inhibit ovulation. The principle of dealing with missed pills is by understanding that seven pills can be omitted without ovulation (as is routinely done in the pill-free week) and that more than seven pills missed in total risks ovulation and thus pregnancy.
- If the pills have been missed after taking seven active tablets, there is a negligible risk of breakthrough ovulation in this case. The woman should be instructed to continue taking the tablets leaving the missed pills. If there are more than seven pills left in the packet she can start her next packet after the pill-free interval or after taking the dummy 'reminder' tablets (in case of 28-day packaging). If there are less than seven pills left however, she should forego the pill-free interval and start her next packet straight away.
- If the tablets have been missed from the beginning of the packet, after the pill-free interval, there is a risk of ovulation due to the effective lengthening of the pill-free interval to 10 days. In this case, emergency contraception should be recommended.
- This can be either in the form of an intrauterine contraceptive device, the progesterone-only pill (Levonelle-2), or the combined oestrogen–progesterone emergency pills.
- In the case of the copper IUD, it should be inserted within 5 days of unprotected intercourse. With the pills, the first should be taken within 72 h of unprotected intercourse. The woman should continue with her regular combined oral contraceptive pill after emergency contraception and use additional barrier methods of contraception for the next 7 days. She should also be instructed to report to her doctor for the exclusion of pregnancy if she has no bleeding in the next pill-free interval.

Q107. A 13-year-old girl comes to you requesting contraception. Her parents are not aware of the fact that she is sexually active. Critically appraise the way that you will approach the problem.

A107.

- The legal age of consent in the UK is 16 years. Though the advantages of delaying sexual intercourse should be put to the girl in an unpatronizing manner, contraception should not be refused as long as the conditions which are described below are fulfilled.
- A medical contraceptive can be prescribed below the age of consent without parental knowledge if the girl understands the doctor's advice;

Fraser comp

cannot be persuaded to inform the parents or allow the doctor to inform them; is very likely to continue to have sexual intercourse with or without contraceptive treatment; her physical or mental health are likely to suffer unless she receives contraceptive advice or treatment; and her best interests require the doctor to proceed without parental consent. All these factors constitute what is termed 'Gillick competence'.

- A modern low dose oestrogen combined pill is usually a suitable method. Injectables and implants are preferable to intrauterine contraceptive devices because of the risk of pelvic infections.
- The importance of the use of condoms, whatever the contraceptive method used, should be stressed because of the risk of sexually transmitted diseases.
- Reliance on the condom alone for contraception should be advised against, and if selected, every opportunity should be taken to mention the emergency pill.

Q108. A woman comes to you wanting to know if the contraceptive implant would be suitable for her. She is a long-standing type I insulin-dependent diabetic, with no immediate plans to conceive. Critically appraise the advice you will give her.

A108.

- The only marketed implant in the UK currently is Implanon, containing 68 mg of etonorgestrel, in the form of a single rod. Its duration of use is typically 3 years, and its efficacy is excellent, acting primarily by ovulation inhibition.
- The advantage of a contraceptive implant in a diabetic is the avoidance of the use of oestrogens. The other progesterone-only methods such as the progesterone-only pill (POP), or the injectables need repeated administration, whereas with Implanon, one subdermal insertion is all that is required for the next 3 years.
- Blood levels are steady rather than fluctuating (POP), or initially too high (injectables). This minimizes metabolic changes, the HDL/LDL lipid ratio remaining unchanged.
- It may alter bleeding patterns, and frequent bleeding or spotting is a disadvantage.
- Contraceptive efficacy may be less in the obese, and it may have to be replaced sooner than 3 years.
- There may be other minor side-effects such as acne, headache, abdominal pain, breast pain, mood changes and gain in weight.

- Discussion of the levonorgestrel intrauterine system should also be done if the POP or injectables are not desired due to the need for repeated administration. This too has a 5-year duration of use, a reduced incidence of pelvic inflammatory disease (significant in diabetics), and excellent contraceptive efficacy, comparable to sterilization.

Chapter 8
Menstrual disorders

Chapter 8: Questions

Answers are on pp. 135–141

Q109. A 32-year-old woman is referred to you by her GP with premenstrual syndrome. Critically appraise how you will proceed to diagnose and treat her.

Q110. A 52-year-old postmenopausal woman presents to the gynaecology clinic with severe postmenopausal vasomotor symptoms. Her GP had suggested that she should start hormone replacement therapy. She is worried because her sister developed extensive deep venous thrombosis while she was taking HRT at the age of 55 years. Outline your assessment of this case.

Q111. Critically appraise the role of selective oestrogen receptor modulators in modern gynaecological practice.

Q112. A 21-year-old woman presents to the gynaecology clinic complaining of severe disabling dysmenorrhoea, which did not respond to conventional analgesics. Justify your management.

Q113. Critically appraise the use of progestogen intrauterine system for the treatment of idiopathic menorrhagia.

Q114. Evaluate the usefulness of add-back therapy along with GnRH analogues.

Q115. A 34-year-old woman is referred to you by her GP with the complaint of chronic pelvic pain. Critically appraise the way you will manage the problem.

Q116. A 51-year-old postmenopausal woman is seeking your advice about her vasomotor symptoms, as well as her worries about developing osteoporosis. She had recently had mastectomy for oestrogen-receptor positive breast cancer. The recommendation of her breast surgeon was not to go on oestrogen replacement therapy. Outline your advice to her.

Q117. You are asked to counsel a 45-year-old woman undergoing a hysterectomy for menorrhagia. She wants to know the pros and cons of having a subtotal operation. She has always had normal cervical smears. Critically appraise the advice you will give her.

Chapter 8: **Answers**

Q109. A 32-year-old woman is referred to you by her GP with premenstrual syndrome. Critically appraise how you will proceed to diagnose and treat her.

A109.

- Premenstrual syndrome is defined as the cyclical occurrence of physical, psychological or behavioural symptoms recurring during the luteal phase of the menstrual cycle and resolving completely by the end of menstruation. There should be a symptom-free week between the end of menstruation and the time of ovulation. The symptoms should be severe enough to interfere with normal functioning or interpersonal relationships.

- It is important to differentiate it from other psychological or physical symptoms. The other fact that is important to ascertain is the degree of symptoms that the woman is suffering.

- The maintenance of a menstrual chart should be recommended in order to reach an accurate diagnosis. The pattern should be repeated in at least four of the previous six cycles.

- In case of doubt about an accurate diagnosis a trial with gonadotrophin-releasing hormone analogue is done. The basis of this test is the assumption that true premenstrual syndrome is due to normal ovarian activity which triggers neuroendocrine activity within the central nervous system. By suppressing this activity with GnRH analogues, premenstrual symptoms should be abolished completely. If symptoms continue, a psychiatric disorder should be suspected.

- GnRH analogues can also be used for treatment of the symptoms of PMS. The side-effects are due to the hypo-oestrogenic state induced by complete suppression of ovarian activity. These include vasomotor symptoms and atrophic vaginitis and more significantly, trabecular bone loss and osteoporosis. These symptoms can be prevented by 'add-back' therapy with tibolone or hormone replacement therapy.

- There is no proven role of progestogens in the treatment of premenstrual syndrome.

- Oestrogenic ovarian suppression can eliminate premenstrual symptoms but as unopposed oestrogen can cause endometrial hyperplasia and cancer it is imperative to deliver progesterone to protect the endometrium. This may reintroduce the symptoms. The answer may be to deliver the oestrogens in the form of patches, implants or gel with local progesterone in the form of the levonorgestrel intrauterine system or progesterone gel.

- Danazol is effective in abolishing symptoms of PMS but it has potential masculinizing effects and induces unfavourable lipid changes. Its side-effects limit the duration of treatment.

- In women who require simultaneous contraception, the combined oral contraceptive pill given without a pill-free interval suppresses ovulation and provides symptomatic relief.
- Selective serotonin reuptake inhibitors are effective in treating behavioural as well as physical symptoms. These act on the principle that altered serotonergic activity occurs in premenstrual syndrome. The most commonly used drug in this category is fluoxetine. Others include sertraline, citalopram and paroxetine.
- In case of extremely severe symptoms of PMS, the only option may remain surgical treatment in the form of a hysterectomy and bilateral salpingo-oophorectomy. This is an extreme step and seldom required. A hysterectomy alone will not resolve the issue and removal of both ovaries becomes mandatory. This should then be followed by oestrogen replacement.

Q110. A 52-year-old postmenopausal woman presents to the gynaecology clinic with severe postmenopausal vasomotor symptoms. Her GP had suggested that she should start hormone replacement therapy. She is worried because her sister developed extensive deep venous thrombosis while she was taking HRT at the age of 55 years. Outline your assessment of this case.

A110.

- The aim of the assessment is to balance the benefits if taking HRT against their risks, particularly in view of the family history of DVT.
- The benefits of HRT are short-term reduction in vasomotor symptoms and urogenital oestrogen deficiency; and long-term reduction in osteoporosis.
- The risks of HRT are the increased risk of DVT (30 vs. 10 : 100 000 women per year) and breast cancer.
- The particular issue here is whether there is increased risk of DVT because of the possibility of increased familial tendency.
- A full personal history of thromboembolic disease and risk factors should be taken. Also, full family history regarding thromboembolic disease.
- Tests for congenital thrombophilia (factor V Leiden mutation, protein C, protein S, antithrombin III, prothrombin 20210 A gene) should be done.
- In the absence of personal or strong family history (two first degree relatives), as well as normal tests, there is no increased risk (over and above that of HRT).

- In the presence of personal history, strong family history or abnormal tests, the risk is increased and HRT is only justified after detailed counselling and risk assessment, ideally involving a thrombophilia expert.

Q111. Critically appraise the role of selective oestrogen receptor modulators in modern gynaecological practice.

A111.

- Selective oestrogen receptor modulators (SERMS) are tamoxifen-related compounds that possess tissue-specific oestrogen agonist and antagonistic effects. Raloxifene is one of the drugs that is licensed for use in the UK. Other drugs include idoxifene and droloxifene, which are currently under development.
- Raloxifene reduces bone loss and thus is indicated for the treatment and prevention of osteoporosis in postmenopausal women. It has been shown to significantly increase bone density at the hip and lumbar spine and reduce bone loss in the proximal femur and total body.
- The relative risk of breast cancer in women treated with these drugs is significantly lower, thus making it ideal for women where HRT is contraindicated due to a history of breast cancer.
- There is no increase in the risk of endometrial cancer or of postmenopausal bleeding with its use.
- It reduces the serum concentrations of total cholesterol and low density lipoproteins while high density lipoproteins and triglycerides remain unchanged, thus reducing the overall risk of cardiovascular disease.
- There is an association with venous thromboembolism, with an incidence of 3.5 per 10 000 users per year.
- Raloxifene use is associated with a small increase in the frequency of hot flushes, leg cramps and peripheral oedema.
- The disadvantage of these agents is that they do not relieve the vasomotor symptoms and psychological disturbances of the menopause. They cannot therefore, fully replace conventional HRT but are a useful substitute in women who want to reduce the risk of osteoporosis and cardiovascular disease while not increasing their risk of breast cancer.

Q112. A 21-year-old woman presents to the gynaecology clinic complaining of severe disabling dysmenorrhoea, which did not respond to conventional analgesics. Justify your management.

A112.

- One should differentiate between primary dysmenorrhoea, which does not have any underlying organic cause, and secondary dysmenorrhoea, which does. This can be initially done by taking a detailed history, physical examination and carrying out an ultrasound scan. If these methods fail, and the condition proves refractory to conventional treatments, consideration should be given to carrying out a diagnostic laparoscopy.
- In case of primary dysmenorrhoea, initial treatment with non-steroidal anti-inflammatory drugs such as mefenamic acid should be tried.
- The combined oral contraceptive pill improves symptoms in up to 80–90% of women with primary dysmenorrhoea.
- The levonorgestrel-releasing intrauterine system causes reduced local prostaglandin production in an atrophic decidualized endometrium. This reduces the pain as well as the bleeding in case of dysfunctional uterine bleeding.
- Secondary dysmenorrhoea can be caused by endometriosis, adenomyosis, fibroids and chronic pelvic inflammatory disease. Treating these will in most cases get rid of the dysmenorrhoea.
- Laparoscopic uterine nerve ablation (LUNA), which involves transection of the uterosacral ligaments and hence of the nerve pathways for pain, may have a role to play in the management of dysmenorrhoea as suggested by early studies.

Q113. Critically appraise the use of progestogen intrauterine system for the treatment of idiopathic menorrhagia.

A113.

- The mode of action of progestogen (P) IUS in idiopathic menorrhagia is suppression of the endometrium.
- The severity of the symptoms must be taken into account when deciding if and what treatment to give (e.g. anaemia, inconvenience, effect on social and professional life). Compared with medical therapy, P-IUS is more likely to lead to amenorrhoea (32%) and has a higher continuation rate (70% vs. 22%) at 3 months of use.
- Compared with endometrial ablation, P-IUS is associated with less mean reduction in menstrual loss, but equal patient satisfaction. Compared with hysterectomy, P-IUS is also associated with equal patient satisfaction, and is more cost-effective
- P-IUS may be considered in women who have failed medical treatment for menorrhagia, but are still considering pregnancy.

- An added advantage is reliable (and reversible) contraception.
- It requires trained staff for insertion and can remain in place for up to 5 years.
- About 20% of women using P-IUS will discontinue its use in the first year because of expulsion, intermenstrual bleeding or spotting.
- All suitable treatment options should be considered and discussed with the patient.

Q114. Evaluate the usefulness of add-back therapy along with GnRH analogues.

A114.

Rationale:

- The side-effects of GnRH-a could be reduced—even prevented—by the concomitant use of add-back HRT.
- These include hot flushes, night sweats, irritability and bone demineralization.

Clinical situations where this use is suitable include:

- Treatment of dysmenorrhoea.
- Endometriosis, as studies have shown the benefits from GnRH-a are not reduced by the use of add-back HRT.

Clinical situations where this use is not suitable include:

- Down-regulation for assisted conception treatment.
- Where a hypo-oestrogenic state is aimed for.
- In the presence of a uterus progestogen should be added to oestrogen in HRT, in an appropriate dose and duration.
- The use of add-back HRT is particularly important when GnRH-a is going to be used for more than 6 months.

Q115. A 34-year-old woman is referred to you by her GP with the complaint of chronic pelvic pain. Critically appraise the way you will manage the problem.

A115.

- A detailed history should be elicited from the patient in order to identify any pathological cause and also to gain the trust and confidence of the patient. Cyclical pain should be distinguished from non-cyclical pain.
- A complete physical examination should then be undertaken with attention to the abdomen, lumbosacral area, and external and internal genital organs. A thorough vaginal examination to elicit any adnexal masses is a must. Genital swabs to rule out pelvic infections should be taken at the

same time. Baseline investigations in the form of a full blood count, ESR, and urine analysis should be performed if not done before.

- Ultrasound is used to confirm the nature of an adnexal mass and identify uterine fibroids as distinguished from ovarian masses.
- The use of laparoscopy is well established in the diagnosis and treatment of conditions associated with chronic pelvic pain. A negative laparoscopy does not imply that there is no physical cause for the pain.
- Medical treatment in the form of danazol, the combined oral contraceptive pill, and GnRH analogues are often of use in the control of symptoms.
- A 'see and treat' approach during laparoscopy can be adopted with prior consent of the woman. Endometriotic lesions as well as pelvic adhesions can be excised. In up to 40% of women who undergo laparoscopy, no cause for pain can be found.
- Presacral neurectomy and laparoscopic uterine nerve ablation techniques may give relief in certain cases.
- In women who opt for hysterectomy with bilateral salpingo-oophorectomy as a last resort, it is important that they are counselled thoroughly prior to surgery about the possibility that their pain will not be cured in spite of it.

Q116. A 51-year-old postmenopausal woman is seeking your advice about her vasomotor symptoms, as well as her worries about developing osteoporosis. She had recently had mastectomy for oestrogen-receptor positive breast cancer. The recommendation of her breast surgeon was not to go on oestrogen replacement therapy. Outline your advice to her.
A116.

Alternatives for the relief of vasomotor symptoms:

- Progestogens, in the form of megestrol acetate in a dose of 40 mg daily or alternatively, medroxyprogesterone acetate can significantly reduce vasomotor symptoms.
- Non-hormonal preparations such as clonidine and propranolol have not been shown to have a significant effect in reducing hot flushes and cause a lot of side-effects.

Alternatives for the prevention of osteoporosis:

- Selective oestrogen receptor modulators (SERMs), such as raloxifene prevents bone loss and increases bone mineral density.
- Other alternatives in the prevention and treatment of osteoporosis include the biphosphonate, etidronate, or alendronate, which reduce bone loss and fracture rates.

- Dietary modification, with the ingestion of 1000–1500 mg of calcium daily, should be encouraged and a reduction in the intake of caffeine, alcohol, salt and animal protein should be encouraged. Calcium supplements are appropriate in those who are unable to modify their diet.
- Lifestyle modification, with reduction in smoking and encouraging weight bearing exercise such as walking.

Q117. You are asked to counsel a 45-year-old woman undergoing a hysterectomy for menorrhagia. She wants to know the pros and cons of having a subtotal operation. She has always had normal cervical smears. Critically appraise the advice you will give her.

A117.

- The subtotal procedure for hysterectomies has come back into focus in recent years mainly due to the success of the cervical screening programme. There are both advantages and disadvantages to the procedure and these need to be thoroughly discussed beforehand with the patient and proper informed consent taken.
- A subtotal hysterectomy takes a shorter operating time, thus reducing the time under anaesthesia as well. As less dissection and bladder mobilization is needed, there is subsequently a lower risk of primary haemorrhage and damage to bladder and ureters.
- Sexual intercourse may be able to be resumed earlier, with better vaginal lubrication possibly being a causative factor.
- The woman needs to be made aware of the continuing need for cervical cytology. There is also a possibility that cervical pathology may develop in the future, with a need for subsequent treatment.
- Some women resume menstruation from remnants of endometrial tissue present in the cervical canal. If this were to occur, one option would be a large loop excision under laparoscopic guidance.
- Careful documentation of the explanations given and the patient's decision should be made in the case notes.

Chapter 9
Urogynaecology

Chapter 9: Questions

Answers are on pp. 144–151

Q118. A 55-year-old woman is diagnosed as having genuine stress incontinence on urodynamic evaluation. She is not keen to undergo surgery. Critically appraise the options you will offer her.

Q119. Critically evaluate the methods used for the management of a case of proven detrusor instability in a postmenopausal woman.

Q120. A 55-year-old woman presents to your clinic complaining of constantly 'being wet' with symptoms of urgency, frequency, nocturia and occasional episodes of haematuria. Critically appraise the investigations you will undertake before planning treatment.

Q121. A 65-year-old woman has been referred to the gynaecology clinic with uterovaginal prolapse. Discuss the factors to be taken into consideration when deciding on the management.

Q122. A woman undergoes a Burch colposuspension for stress incontinence. Following this, she is unable to void urine. Critically appraise the steps you will undertake to manage this situation.

Q123. A 45-year-old woman presents to your clinic complaining of faecal incontinence. The problem has gradually worsened over time but she has been too embarrassed to consult a doctor. Critically appraise your management of the condition.

Q124. A woman undergoes an abdominal hysterectomy for extensive endometriosis. She presents 2 weeks later with the complaint of 'continuous urinary incontinence'. How will you reach a diagnosis? Justify your management in this case.

Q125. A woman undergoes a Wertheim's hysterectomy. In the postoperative period she develops a pyrexia, flank pain and persistent haematuria. You suspect ureteric injury. Critically appraise the steps you will undertake to reach a diagnosis and institute a plan of management.

Q126. A 60-year-old woman is referred by her GP with the complaint of 'something coming down in the vagina' as well as feeling a lump. She underwent a hysterectomy for menorrhagia at the age of 45 years. Justify your management.

Q127. Evaluate methods of preventing enterocoele occurrence following operative gynaecological procedures.

Chapter 9: **Answers**

Q118. A 55-year-old woman is diagnosed as having genuine stress incontinence on urodynamic evaluation. She is not keen to undergo surgery. Critically appraise the options you will offer her.
A118.
- There are several options of conservative management for genuine stress incontinence. The advantages are the lack of morbidity associated with surgery and also the satisfaction rate, which can be quite high for individual patients.
- The modification of fluid intake often reduces symptoms of incontinence. This is aided by the maintenance of a frequency–volume chart. Other measures which may help are the treatment of chronic coughs or constipation which may worsen symptoms as well as the reduction of weight.
- Bladder retraining has been shown to be effective in controlling symptoms. Voiding on schedule and relaxation techniques to suppress urge sensations are taught.
- Physiotherapy in the form of pelvic floor exercises to strengthen the pelvic floor muscles which support the bladder can give up to a 60% improvement at 5 years follow-up.
- Vaginal cones can be used as adjuncts to pelvic floor exercises to treat the symptoms of stress incontinence. They are used in gradually increasing weights to be retained in the vagina by both passive and active contraction of the pelvic floor muscles.
- Electrical pudendal nerve stimulation with electrodes placed in the vagina or anus is used to augment urethral sphincteric function and inhibit bladder contractility. It has been shown to have some success in controlling symptoms, though not as much as physiotherapy.
- Oestrogens have not been conclusively shown to have a beneficial effect on the symptoms of stress incontinence.
- Mechanical devices to elevate and support the bladder neck or to occlude the urethra are used to treat the symptoms of incontinence. These include intravaginal continence guards, which elevate the bladder neck. Urethral devices include urethral plugs, suction cups, urethral inserts and continence control pads.

Q119. Critically evaluate the methods used for the management of a case of proven detrusor instability in a postmenopausal woman.
A119.
- Detrusor instability (DI) is a chronic problem that usually requires long-term treatment, multidisciplinary input and active patient involvement.

- General measures: explanation to patient, fluid restriction to 1.5 L daily, avoidance of caffeine (diuretic and detrusor stimulant), and treatment of urinary infection if present.
- Bladder retraining: requires committed and compliant patient and an experienced team. Of proven short-term benefit but no data on long-term results nor on outcome in combination with drugs.
- Physiotherapy: of benefit in cases of mixed incontinence in combination with bladder drill. Careful supervision and instructions are essential.
- Anticholinergic drugs: oxybutinin and tolterodine. Discussion should include dosage, side-effects, results and different formulae (i.e. modified-release).
- Tricyclic antidepressants and DDAVP in nocturnal enuresis.
- HRT: of no proven benefit.
- Surgical management: transvesical phenol injection, bladder transection or distension are of no proven benefit. Augmentation 'clam' cystoplasty is used in intractable cases with incapacitating symptoms and no adequate response to other measures.

Q120. A 55-year-old woman presents to your clinic complaining of constantly 'being wet' with symptoms of urgency, frequency, nocturia and occasional episodes of haematuria. Critically appraise the investigations you will undertake before planning treatment.
A120.

- A mid-stream specimen of urine should be taken for culture and sensitivity to rule out a urinary tract infection as this often gives rise to the above symptoms.
- A frequency–volume chart should be maintained by the patient to give an idea about fluid intake and voiding patterns as well as episodes of incontinence and whether these were precipitated by urgency or activity.
- Uroflowmetry, to measure the urinary flow rate in order to rule out voiding problems should be undertaken prior to urodynamic assessment.
- Cystometry should always be performed where there are multiple symptoms of urge and stress incontinence with frequency. They should also be carried out for voiding disorders, prior to any bladder neck surgery and in neuropathic bladder disorders. Twin channel cystometry is the most commonly used method.
- The ambulatory urodynamic method is a more physiological way of monitoring and thus a more accurate way of reaching a diagnosis.

UTI
Bladder stone
Tumor
neuropathic

- In view of the symptoms of haematuria, a cystourethroscopy should be undertaken to rule out the presence of calculus or a bladder tumour. It can be performed under a general or local anaesthetic.
- Ultrasound is a non-invasive method of checking residual urinary volume, as well as bladder wall thickness.
- Videocystourethrography is radiological screening of the bladder synchronized with pressure studies. It is done in patients complaining of postmicturition dribble due to diverticulae, ureteric reflux or in the investigation of a neuropathic bladder. It is not a routine part of the investigations for incontinence.

Q121. A 65-year-old woman has been referred to the gynaecology clinic with uterovaginal prolapse. Discuss the factors to be taken into consideration when deciding on the management.
A121.
- Extent of prolapse and symptoms caused.
- Impact on quality of life.
- Social situation (e.g. looking after elderly partner).
- Associated urinary or bowel symptoms.
- The presence of other genital pathology.
- General health and other illnesses (aggravating symptoms such as cough/ fitness for GA).
- The woman's wishes regarding retaining a functional vagina.
- The woman's wishes for treatment.

Q122. A woman undergoes a Burch colposuspension for stress incontinence. Following this, she is unable to void urine. Critically appraise the steps you will undertake to manage this situation.
A122.
- A catheter should be inserted to prevent bladder over-distension and a CSU should be checked to rule out a urinary tract infection.
- It is important to ensure that the patient is not constipated and is mobile after surgery.
- If the problem persists after surgery, urodynamic investigations should be carried out to try to elucidate the cause of the problem.
- Pharmacological treatments in the form of acetylcholine inhibitors such as distigmine bromide, cholinergic agonists such as bethanocol chloride or α-adrenergic blocking agents have not been shown to have a significant effect on the problem.

- Surgical treatment involves urethral dilatation, Otis urethrotomy or endoscopic bladder neck incision. Care should be taken to avoid over-dilatation, and to minimize the risk of producing sphincter weakness or incontinence.
- If surgery does not help to overcome the voiding difficulties, then clean intermittent self-catheterization (CISC) should be used. Patients should be counselled regarding its use which will aid in acceptance of the technique. It is associated with the risk of repeated urinary tract infections which should be looked for and treated.

Q123. A 45-year-old woman presents to your clinic complaining of faecal incontinence. The problem has gradually worsened over time but she has been too embarrassed to consult a doctor. Critically appraise your management of the condition.

A123.

- A detailed history is essential including duration of symptoms, frequency of incontinent episodes, and severity which is graded according to loss of control for flatus, liquid or solid stool. Coexisting symptoms of urinary incontinence should be asked for. The presence of neurological symptoms are ascertained and history of vaginal deliveries including the use of forceps and occurrence of perineal tears as well as any previous surgery to the anal canal and gastrointestinal tract such as anal dilatation should be taken.
- A thorough examination includes a general examination as well as inspection of the perineum which may reveal faecal soiling, perianal excoriation, fistulae, scars from previous perianal sepsis, tears or episiotomy. A digital examination should be carried out to examine the internal anal and voluntary sphincter function.
- Proctoscopy and sigmoidoscopy can be carried out at the first visit, especially where mucosal prolapse is suspected.
- Disruption of the anal sphincter muscles is best assessed by anal ultrasound examination. In certain cases, MRI may be useful.
- Surgical repair in case of disruption of the anal sphincter should be undertaken by a person experienced in the technique. In the case of extensive muscle loss, a defunctioning colostomy may be required. The external anal sphincter is mobilized widely and the cut ends are sutured end to end or in an overlapping manner with non-absorbable monofilament sutures.
- In the case of rectal mucosal prolapse causing incontinence, rubber band ligation or injections with sclerosants can be done. Alternatively, a

Perineal tears
anal / GI surg.
neuropathie
rectal mucosal prolapse

perineal or abdominal approach to correction of the prolapse is undertaken. The rectum is mobilized and fixed to the sacrum by sutures or
a mesh.

- Biofeedback training, where the patients are taught to recognize rectal
distension and to contract their voluntary sphincters may play a role in
the control of symptoms.

Q124. A woman undergoes an abdominal hysterectomy for extensive
endometriosis. She presents 2 weeks later with the complaint of 'continuous urinary incontinence'. How will you reach a diagnosis? Justify your
management in this case.

A124.

- The specific complaint of continuously leaking urine postoperatively is
usually associated with the occurrence of a urogenital fistula. It typically
presents 7–14 days postoperatively.
- The investigation of first choice is to carry out dye studies. Methylene
blue is instilled into the bladder with the patient in lithotomy. Any
leakage is directly visualized. Any staining of a tampon placed in the
vagina will reveal a vesicovaginal fistula. The 'three' swab test is not
recommended as it gives a less clear distinction between urethral and
extra-urethral leakage, as also the identification of multiple fistulae.
If leakage of fluid continues after instillation of the dye, a ureteric
fistula is likely. A 'two dye test' using phenazopyridine to stain the
renal urine and methylene blue to stain the bladder contents can be
used.
- Intravenous urography is done to rule out any damage to the upper
urinary tract.
- A careful examination under anaesthesia is done, not only to ascertain the
site of the fistula, but also to decide the route of surgical approach
needed, whether vaginal or abdominal.
- A cystourethroscopy is performed at the same time to determine the exact
position and level of the fistula in relation to the ureteric orifices and
bladder neck.
- Catheterization should be carried out. This sometimes will lead to spontaneous resolution of the fistula, and a trial of 6–8 weeks should be given
before doing a surgical repair. This will also allow for any slough to
separate and inflammatory changes to resolve.
- The route of surgical repair, whether abdominal or vaginal, is decided by
the access and mobility of vaginal tissue. Interposition grafting by muscle,
peritoneum or omentum in an abdominal approach, or a Martius graft of

dye studies   CSU
IVU   catheterisation ~2wks
EUA
Cystourethroscopy

labial fat and bulbocavernosus muscle in the vaginal approach, is used to reinforce the repair.

- Continuous bladder drainage in the postoperative period is imperative. Both the urethral or suprapubic route, alone or together, can be used. It should remain *in situ* for at least 2 weeks.

Q125. A woman undergoes a Wertheim's hysterectomy. In the postoperative period she develops a pyrexia, flank pain and persistent haematuria. You suspect ureteric injury. Critically appraise the steps you will undertake to reach a diagnosis and institute a plan of management.

A125.

- The ureters can be injured near the pelvic brim in gynaecological surgery, where they lie adjacent to the ovarian vessels or low down beside the cervix, where they are crossed by the uterine vessels. They can either be crushed in clamps or included in ligatures.
- It is important to define the precise nature of the ureteric injury. A catheter specimen of urine should be taken for culture and sensitivity. Blood urea and serum electrolytes should be checked routinely and dehydration or electrolyte imbalance should be corrected.
- An intravenous urogram should be carried out. This will reveal obstruction at the site of injury. High dose intravenous urograms with delayed films will show the level of the site of injury by showing the lower limit of the intact ureter.
- Cystoscopy will reveal the side of the affected ureter as there will be no efflux of urine from that ureteric orifice. Indigo carmine may be used.
- Percutaneous nephrostomy under ultrasound control and descending ureterography or alternatively cystoscopy with ascending ureterography will delineate the level of the injury.
- Once the nature of the lesion has been defined, a decision should be made about the method of treatment. In early cases, simple ureteric drainage with a double J stent may allow a small fistula to heal.
- If the ureter is completely obstructed, reconstruction or reimplantation should be undertaken. There is a risk of stricture formation with the latter. Direct reimplantation can be done by using a psoas hitch, or the creation of a flap of bladder wall (Boari–Ockerblad technique). Where there is significant deficiency, the ureter may have to be transplanted into the opposite ureter, a ureteroureterostomy or to interpose a loop of small bowel.

Q126. A 60-year-old woman is referred by her GP with the complaint of 'something coming down in the vagina' as well as feeling a lump. She underwent a hysterectomy for menorrhagia at the age of 45 years. Justify your management.

A126.

- The most likely diagnosis in this case is that of a vaginal vault prolapse following a hysterectomy. It is important to delineate the extent of the prolapse and to identify any coexisting urinary or bowel symptoms before embarking on surgery.
- A detailed history and examination should be undertaken. Urinary and bowel symptoms should be asked for, including the presence of incontinence, and investigated if present. The extent of the vault prolapse, along with the existence of a cystocoele, rectocoele or enterocoele should be noted.
- In order to prevent recurrence and ensure a successful surgical outcome, preoperative weight reduction and improvement of chronic chest conditions should be undertaken. Use of topical oestrogen preparations and treatment of dependent ulceration facilitates surgery.
- Colporrhaphy, i.e. anterior and posterior vaginal repair along with obliteration of the enterocoele sac alone is not adequate for the treatment of significant vault prolapse.
- Transvaginal sacrospinous colpopexy, where the vaginal vault is fixed to the sacrospinous ligament via a transvaginal approach, has up to a 95% success rate. If a cystocoele is present, it is repaired first, followed by an anterior vaginal repair with suburethral buttressing sutures. This is followed by the sacrospinous colpopexy.
- Alternatively, an abdominal sacral colpopexy, involving the suspension of the vaginal vault from the sacral promontory using a synthetic mesh (mersilene or Teflon) is used. Coexisting cystocoele or rectocoele are repaired vaginally first. Patients should be warned of the risks of intraoperative haemorrhage and infection of the mesh.
- A synchronous abdominoperineal procedure can also be done. However, this is a more complicated procedure, with a lower success rate than sacral colpopexy.
- Coexisting symptoms of stress incontinence are treated by a bladder neck suspension procedure such as the tension-free vaginal tape along with a sacrospinous colpopexy. Alternatively, a Burch colposuspension with an abdominal vault supporting procedure can be carried out.
- Marked rectal prolapse along with vault prolapse can be treated by a postanal sacrorectopexy in addition to sacrospinous colpopexy.

Q127. Evaluate methods of preventing enterocoele occurrence following operative gynaecological procedures.

A127.

- Conservative measures of preventing enterocoele formation are encouraging weight loss prior to surgery and maintaining this postoperatively. Topical and systemic oestrogens should be used to improve tissues and treat dependent ulcers. Chronic cough or constipation should be treated, and patients dissuaded from smoking. Pelvic floor exercises will help in maintaining the tone of the pelvic floor.

- At the time of vaginal hysterectomy, a 'culdoplasty', where a delayed absorption suture is used to bring the two uterosacral ligaments together after obliterating the enterocoele sac and plicating them to the vaginal vault, is a valuable method of preventing enterocoele.

- Sacrospinous colpopexy, done after a vaginal hysterectomy, can prevent vault prolapse and is a treatment for enterocoele formation. It has up to a 92% success rate.

- Procedures after abdominal surgery include sacrocolpopexy, where the vaginal vault is suspended from the sacral promontory by a mesh (dacron/Teflon), and the posterior peritoneum is closed over this. This can be done via the laparoscopic route too.

- A Moschowitz procedure, where circular sutures are used to obliterate the pouch of Douglas, can also be used. Abdominoperineal repair, where both the abdominal and vaginal routes are used simultaneously, is another procedure with a success rate only slightly lower than sacrospinous fixation.

Chapter 10
Gynaecological emergencies and benign conditions

Chapter 10: Questions

Answers are on pp. 154–165

Q128. A healthy young woman has had three pregnancies, all of which ended in spontaneous miscarriage at 10–12 weeks gestation. Evaluate the tests available for determining a cause for her recurrent pregnancy loss.

Q129. A woman presents at 8 weeks gestation requesting a termination of pregnancy. How will you manage the case, what are the particular risks involved, and how will you avoid them?

Q130. A 25-year-old woman with a history of primary infertility has a tubal pregnancy. She is haemodynamically stable. Debate the options available for the treatment of her ectopic pregnancy.

Q131. A 28-year-old woman presents to the gynaecology clinic complaining of recurrent vulvovaginal candidiasis. Critically appraise how you will go about treating her.

Q132. How can you improve and maintain the quality of care provided by your department to patients in your hospital?

Q133. A 5-year-old girl is brought to your gynaecology clinic by her mother who is very worried about a vaginal discharge that the girl has been getting for the past few days. How will you go about diagnosing and treating the condition?

Q134. Critically appraise the possible complications of hysteroscopic surgery and how to avoid them.

Q135. While carrying out a transcervical resection of the endometrium (TCRE), the surgeon is informed by the scrub nurse that there is a deficit in the fluid output as compared to the input. What should be the optimal management of such a case?

Q136. A perforation is suspected while undertaking a hysteroscopic myomectomy. Critically appraise your management.

Q137. A woman is readmitted to hospital at 8 weeks gestation with severe hyperemesis gravidarum. This is her third admission to hospital in the past 2 weeks. Critically appraise your management.

Q138. Laparoscopy is occasionally associated with bowel damage. How may this risk be minimized and how may such damage be recognized?

Q139. You are called to see a 27-year-old woman who has presented with acute pelvic pain to the A & E department. She had a normal menstrual period 10 days ago. A urine pregnancy test is negative. The surgeons have seen her and provisionally ruled out a surgical cause for the pain. Critically appraise your approach to her management.

Q140. You are asked to deal with an 18-year-old female victim of rape who has presented to the hospital. In the absence of a forensic physician, you are asked to examine her. Critically appraise the steps you will take.

Q141. An 18-year-old girl complains of a vaginal discharge and has triple swabs taken which are reported positive for *Chlamydia*. Critically appraise how you will counsel and treat the girl.

Chapter 10: **Answers**

Q128. A healthy young woman has had three pregnancies, all of which ended in spontaneous miscarriage at 10–12 weeks gestation. Evaluate the tests available for determining a cause for her recurrent pregnancy loss.
A128.

- Evaluate means to attach a degree of importance to each test. It is similarly important to recognize the negative value of commonly used but outmoded tests.
- The most common cause is PCO. Therefore, the two most important tests are ultrasound scanning of the ovaries and mid-follicular LH/FSH.
- Next in order are the antiphospholipids: lupus anticoagulant and anticardiolipin antibodies.
- The following are important tests for less common causes: karyotyping of both patient and partner, exclusion of uterine abnormality (would be most unusual to remain undiscovered after three miscarriages), thrombophilic profile, especially APCR (this is much more important in second trimester loss) and other immunological tests.
- It is important to mention that tests for metabolic disease such as diabetes and thyroid disease are not necessary as primary tests. Similarly tests for infection such as CMV, toxoplasmosis, *Listeria*, etc. are unnecessary.

Q129. A woman presents at 8 weeks gestation requesting a termination of pregnancy. How will you manage the case, what are the particular risks involved, and how will you avoid them?
A129.

- In the case of a woman requesting a termination, it is important to treat the patient with sympathy and respect. Those women who need more support in decision making should be identified, and facilities for additional support including access to social services should be available.
- Conventional suction termination is an appropriate method at this gestation.
- Cervical priming should be carried out prior to surgery. This can be done with gemeprost 1 mg vaginally 3 h prior to surgery.
- Alternatively, misoprostol 400 µg vaginally 3 h prior to surgery can be used.
- A third method of cervical priming is the use of mifeprestone 200 mg orally 36 h prior to surgery.
- Medical abortion, using mifeprestone 600 mg orally, followed 36–48 h later by gemeprost 1 mg vaginally, or mifeprestone 200 mg orally, followed by misoprostol 800 µg vaginally, can be used.

- In the case of medical abortions, it is important to warn the woman that she may bleed, and prescribe analgesia.
- The main complication at the time of abortion is haemorrhage, which may be reduced with oxytocic drugs.
- Uterine perforation is not common with an incidence of 1–4/1000. It can be avoided by cervical priming prior to surgery and the performance of the procedure by a fully trained and experienced surgeon. In case of suspected uterine perforation, a laparoscopy should be carried out, followed by a laparotomy if necessary.
- Genital tract infections can occur in up to 10% of cases. This can be avoided by taking swabs at the time of the procedure and administering metronidazole 1 g rectally at the time of the procedure. Additionally, doxycycline 100 mg twice daily, should be commenced for a week.

Q130. A 25-year-old woman with a history of primary infertility has a tubal pregnancy. She is haemodynamically stable. Debate the options available for the treatment of her ectopic pregnancy.

A130.

- Management is dependent upon gestational age and trophoblastic activity.
- In the presence of low or falling β-hCG levels, and in an asymptomatic patient, expectant management should be considered.
- Medical treatment with methotrexate is possible:
  with an unruptured ectopic
  in a haemodynamically stable patient
  where the patient is reliable and compliant
  and followed by sequential β-hCG.
- Laparotomy is still the most common approach but laparoscopic treatment is possible.
- The disadvantages of laparoscopic treatment are:
  the inherent dangers of minimal access surgery
  the availability of surgical expertise and suitable equipment
  patient's physical condition
  location, size and state of ectopic.
- The advantages of laparoscopic treatment are:
  shorter hospital stay
  quicker return to normal activities
  less postoperative analgesia
  ?reduction in cost

- Whether laparotomy or laparoscopy is utilized, the surgical options are
salpingectomy
fimbrial expression
linear salpingotomy
segmental excision and reanastomosis.

Q131. A 28-year-old woman presents to the gynaecology clinic complaining of recurrent vulvovaginal candidiasis. Critically appraise how you will go about treating her?
A131.
- Recurrent vulvovaginal candidiasis is defined as four or more mycologically proven episodes of vulvovaginal candidiasis in 1 year.
- It is important to firstly reach an accurate diagnosis. This is done by taking a careful history, including any precipitating causes. The use of long-term antibiotics should be asked for, including the presence of any immune deficiencies such as HIV infection, use of corticosteroids and cytotoxic therapy. Diabetes mellitus is a common cause, as well as the use of combined oral contraceptives and hormone replacement therapy.
- Clinical examination and microbiological investigations including vulval, low vaginal and high vaginal swabs to confirm the presence of candidal infection along with the particular strain of the yeast, and also to rule out other conditions such as bacterial vaginosis, trichomonal vulvovaginitis and wart virus infections should be undertaken. If no diagnosis is apparent, the patient should be asked to attend the clinic when she has a typical recurrence.
- History of the use and duration of antifungal treatment should be taken, as often these women have had short courses of antifungals, with a subsequent exacerbation on discontinuing treatment.
- An intensive course of treatment with topical as well as vaginal pessaries or of oral preparations should be used, followed by maintenance therapy with once weekly fluconazole or clotrimazole vaginal pessaries. Alternatively, daily ketoconazole or itraconazole should be used.
- There is no evidence to prove that simultaneous treatment of the sexual partner is of benefit.

Q132. How can you improve and maintain the quality of care provided by your department to patients in your hospital?

A132.

- The use of evidence-based clinical guidelines to inform health-care professionals about evidence-based practice for discrete clinical topics. These are systematically developed statements which assist clinicians and patients in making decisions about appropriate treatment for specific conditions.
- Education and training to bring such information to the attention of clinicians and health service managers.
- Clinical audit to monitor practice and to promote change where indicated. This is a clinically led initiative which seeks to improve the quality and outcome of patient care. It involves structured peer review whereby clinicians examine their practices and results against agreed standards, and modify their practice where indicated.
- The principle of clinical risk management which involves methods for the early identification of adverse events, using either staff reports or systematic screening of records. This should be followed by creation of a database to identify common patterns and develop a system of accountability to prevent future incidents.
- The use of proper complaints procedures: must be accessible to patients and their families and be fair to staff. Lessons from the analysis of each complaint are learned and the recurrence of similar problems are hopefully avoided.
- Multidisciplinary approach.

Q133. A 5-year-old girl is brought to your gynaecology clinic by her mother who is very worried about a vaginal discharge that the girl has been getting for the past few days. How will you go about diagnosing and treating the condition?

A133.

- A careful history should be taken from the mother and the clinician must gain the child's trust by creating a non-threatening atmosphere. The history must include the duration and frequency of symptoms, the colour and quantity of the discharge and the presence of any odour. As the commonest cause is due to poor local hygiene, detailed questioning about urinary and bowel habits is important including genital cleaning. History of genital manipulation, which is common in young girls and may lead to bacterial transmission to the vulva, should be taken.
- Examination of the child must be undertaken with great care and sensitivity in the presence of the mother. Inspection of the vulva including the

labia, hymen, lower vagina and anus should be done. The possibility of
✗ sexual abuse should be borne in mind and the hymen inspected for any
tears or loss of shape. An aspirate should be obtained for culture using a
pipette and saline, avoiding contact with the child. If there is a suspicion
of a foreign body, a vaginoscopy under an anaesthetic should be considered.

- A majority of cases are due to non-specific vulvovaginitis which may
  cause erythema, vulval pain, excoriation and vaginal discharge. Antibiotics do not have a role in these cases and instructions should be given in
  proper hygiene and care in cleaning the vulva after micturition and
  defecation. Barrier creams may be used and in refractory cases, a short
  course of oestrogen cream may be recommended though this should not
  be used for longer periods because of systemic absorption.
- Specific vulvovaginitis may be caused by various organisms, commonly
  following respiratory infections due to spread of these organisms by the
  child's fingers. These are *Haemophilus influenzae*, group A β-haemolytic
  Streptococcus, *Strep. pneumoniae* and enterobacteria. If culture of the
  discharge reveals any of these infections, antibiotics should be prescribed
  according to sensitivities.
- It is very important to bear in mind the possibility of sexual abuse in
  young children with a discharge. Culture of sexually transmitted organisms such as *Neisseria gonorrhoea*, *Trichomonas vaginalis*, *Chlamydia
  trachomatis*, herpes simplex and human papilloma virus (condyloma
  acuminata) should trigger such a suspicion and these cases should immediately be reported to the proper authorities. There is a possibility of
  digital transmission of *Chlamydia trachomatis* via ocular infections in
  children and this fact should be kept in mind. All the other organisms
  listed above are transmitted via the sexual route. They should be treated
  with the appropriate antibiotics.
- In the case of foreign bodies in the vagina, removal should be carried out
  under an anaesthetic.

Q134. Critically appraise the possible complications of hysteroscopic surgery and how to avoid them.
A134.

- Endometrial thinning with GnRH analogues should be undertaken prior
  to procedures such as endometrial ablation in order to reduce fluid
  absorption and the risk of perforation.
- The hysteroscope should always be introduced under direct vision and the
  ostia identified prior to endometrial ablation. The resection should stop

at the internal os as there is a risk of haemorrhage if resecting into the cervical canal.

- Fluid overload is one of the possible complications of operating hysteroscopy. This can lead to dilutional hyponatraemia and hypokalaemia, which may in turn cause cardiac arrhythmias, cerebral oedema, coma and death. Volume expansion may lead to pulmonary oedema. It is imperative that at all times a record of volume infused and that returned is kept. A 'Hysteromat' can be used for this purpose. If a deficit is found in fluid returned, the operation should be immediately stopped and the problem dealt with.
- Electrolyte-free solution such as glycine should be used in electrosurgery.
- Uterine perforation may occur in 1–2% of cases. It can be very serious, especially if it occurs with the active electrode. If it is suspected, an immediate laparotomy should be performed. In the case of visceral damage to bowel, a laparotomy by an experienced bowel surgeon should be performed and the injury repaired.
- Haemorrhage may complicate 1–3% of cases. If bleeding vessels are identified, they should be coagulated. If uncontrolled, a Foley balloon should be inserted into the uterus and distended with 20–30 mL of saline to create a tamponade.
- One of the possible complications of the procedure is infection which can be prevented by covering all patients with antibiotics at the time of the operation.
- It should be stressed to patients that contraception should be continued after the procedure as it does not guarantee sterility and there is an increased risk of miscarriage, intrauterine growth restriction, and problems with placentation if a pregnancy were to occur.
- It is imperative to sample the endometrium prior to the procedure to rule out the presence of endometrial cancer.

Q135. While carrying out a transcervical resection of the endometrium (TCRE), the surgeon is informed by the scrub nurse that there is a deficit in the fluid output as compared to the input. What should be the optimal management of such a case?

A135.

- Fluid is infused into the uterine cavity under pressure in procedures such as TCRE in order to distend the uterus and maintain a clear operative view. This can be absorbed systemically, with catastrophic consequences if a tab is not kept on the amount infused and that returned.

- The fluid deficit should be accurately measured using a Hysteromat. If this is less than 1000 mL, surgery can be continued, ensuring that no further deficit occurs.
- If the fluid deficit is between 1000 and 1500 mL, the surgery should be expedited. If the fluid absorption increases beyond this, the surgery should be immediately stopped, and the anaesthetist informed of this complication.
- Pulmonary oedema may occur because of volume expansion and a chest X-ray should be undertaken. Frusemide, in the dose of 40 mg, should be given intravenously.
- An indwelling catheter should be inserted and strict input–output monitoring done.
- Urea and electrolytes should be estimated and corrected as dilutional hyponatraemia and hypokalaemia may occur, leading to cardiac arrhythmia and cerebral oedema. An electrocardiogram should be done if this is suspected, and expert medical advice sought.
- The patient must be observed in hospital until her condition settles. A detailed explanation should be given by the consultant-in-charge before discharge.

Q136. A perforation is suspected while undertaking a hysteroscopic myomectomy. Critically appraise your management.

A136.

- Uterine perforation may complicate 1–2% of cases of operative hysteroscopy. If such a case is suspected, the consultant gynaecologist and anaesthetist should be informed.
- If perforation has occurred at the end of the procedure, while retrieving tissue and is not associated with significant bleeding, it can be managed conservatively with observation and antibiotics. The patient should be kept in hospital overnight, and if her situation deteriorates, she should be taken back to theatre.
- If significant haemorrhage occurs, or perforation with the active electrode is suspected, an immediate laparoscopy should be undertaken to assess the damage. Bleeding can be controlled by suturing or diathermy.
- If bowel injury has occurred, a laparotomy by an experienced bowel surgeon should be undertaken. Depending upon the extent of injury, either suturing a perforation, or a resection or anastomosis, with or without a colostomy may be required.
- Uterine perforation at hysteroscopic myomectomy may increase the chances of uterine rupture during the third trimester. These serosal defects

should be sutured, and the patient observed closely in a subsequent pregnancy. Elective caesarean section may be considered in such a case.
- Even if managed conservatively, close observation in hospital is mandatory, as sometimes diathermy injuries to the bowel may go unnoticed, and
✱ present with peritonitis some days later.
- The patient should be informed of events prior to discharge.

Q137. A woman is readmitted to hospital at 8 weeks gestation with severe hyperemesis gravidarum. This is her third admission to hospital in the past 2 weeks. Critically appraise your management.
A137.
- Though hyperemesis gravidarum is a common complaint, it can be associated with severe morbidity and even mortality in those who are seriously affected. It therefore needs to be treated appropriately.
- Other conditions which cause nausea and vomiting need to be ruled out. These include urinary tract infections, peptic ulceration and pancreatitis. Abdominal pain will be a significant feature in these conditions.
- The most important aspect of management is to [restore the fluid and electrolyte imbalance caused.] This should be done by the infusion of normal saline or Hartmann's solution with the addition of potassium chloride as required.
- Dextrose-containing fluids should not be used as they can precipitate
✱ Wernicke's encephalopathy. Double strength saline should also be avoided.
- A fluid balance chart should be maintained and any weight loss recorded on a weekly basis.
- Frequent electrolyte estimations to look for hyponatraemia, hypokalaemia and metabolic hypochloraemic alkalosis should be done. There may be deranged liver function tests in up to 50% of cases.
- Thyroid function tests are usually abnormal in severe cases and do not require treatment, resolving spontaneously when the condition is treated.
- Thiamine deficiency may occur in severe hyperemesis gravidarum and if untreated could lead to Wernicke's encephalopathy. This is characterized by diplopia, abnormal ocular movements, ataxia and confusion. To prevent this, thiamine supplementation, either orally or in the form of weekly intravenous injections should be given.
- Antiemetics in the form of dopamine antagonists, phenothiazines or antihistamines can be safely given.
- Corticosteroids may play a role in those unresponsive to conventional supportive therapy. They should be reduced slowly.

- There may be psychological problems underlying the condition. It is thus imperative that emotional support, reassurance and encouragement should be offered to the patient.
- Total parenteral nutrition may be required in certain extreme cases.

Q138. Laparoscopy is occasionally associated with bowel damage. How may this risk be minimized and how may such damage be recognized?
A138.

General points:
- The risk of bowel damage with laparoscopic surgery is 1 : 500.
- The risk is increased if there is a history of abdominal surgery or previous pelvic inflammatory disease.

Minimizing risk:
- Careful patient selection.
- Appropriate training in operative technique: attainment of laparoscopic training up to appropriate 'skill levels'.
- Correct direction of insertion of instruments.
- Use of guarded point instruments.
- Insertion of subsequent portals under direct vision.
- Use of alternative insertion points for Veress needle if anterior abdominal wall adhesions are suspected such as 'Palmers' point'.

Recognizing damage:
- Difficult if the injured area is empty or not under direct vision.
- Deterioration of condition postoperatively, especially the presence of excessive abdominal or shoulder tip pain, tachycardia, pyrexia or peritoneal irritation.
- The opinion of a bowel surgeon may be helpful, and an exploratory laparotomy essential.

Q139. You are called to see a 27-year-old woman who has presented with acute pelvic pain to the A & E department. She had a normal menstrual period 10 days ago. A urine pregnancy test is negative. The surgeons have seen her and provisionally ruled out a surgical cause for the pain. Critically appraise your approach to her management.
A139.

- Acute pelvic pain may be an indicator of various pathological processes and thus a systematic approach is necessary.
- A detailed history of the exact location, mode of onset and radiation of the pain should be taken. History of pyrexia, vaginal discharge, previous

fibroids, any past abdominal or pelvic operations, and associated symptoms such as nausea, vomiting, diarrhoea, dysuria, frequency or haematuria should be noted.

- A detailed general, abdominal and pelvic examination should be done with consent. Bimanual pelvic examination is done to assess the uterus and adnexa for enlargement or tenderness. High and low vaginal and endocervical swabs are taken. A rectal examination must be performed. Primary investigations include a mid-stream sample of urine for culture and sensitivity, full blood count including a differential count.

- The commonest gynaecological cause of acute pelvic pain is acute pelvic inflammatory disease. Salpingitis usually gives rise to bilateral pelvic pain with pyrexia and vaginal discharge. A frequent cause is chlamydial infection, followed by *Neisseria gonorrhoea*, bacterial vaginosis and others. A previous history of sexually transmitted infections, use of the intrauterine contraceptive device or termination of pregnancy are significant. Antibiotic treatment should be prompt, as it can cause severe morbidity ✳ and infertility later on, if untreated. Tubo-ovarian abscesses will need a laparoscopy with excision and drainage and a prolonged course of antibiotic treatment.

- Torsion of cysts may present with acute pelvic pain. An ultrasound scan should be done to exclude any adnexal masses. If present, a laparoscopy may be needed, followed by a salpingo-oophorectomy or in certain cases where it is feasible and ovarian conservation is desired, detorsion of the ischaemic adnexa.

- Mid-cycle ovulatory pains may give rise to sudden onset, sharp, lower abdominal pain, followed by several hours of dull aching. Conservative management with non-steroidal anti-inflammatory agents and other analgesics is advised.

- Necrosis in fibroids can appear as constant or colicky acute pelvic pain, sometimes with pyrexia. There may be a history of fibroids, and an ultrasound scan will help in diagnosing the condition. Conservative management is usually instituted until the acute episode has resolved. Later, definitive surgery in the form of myomectomy or hysterectomy is undertaken.

Q140. You are asked to deal with an 18-year-old female victim of rape who has presented to the hospital. In the absence of a forensic physician, you are asked to examine her. Critically appraise the steps you will take.

A140.

- The rape victim must be dealt with in a sensitive manner, keeping in mind that she may be in a state of shock from her ordeal. Express permission must be taken, not only to examine her, but also to inform the police. If she does not wish to do so, her wishes have to be respected. A thorough and systematic examination and recording of findings must be done, as they may be used as evidence in any subsequent investigations.
- Written consent to the examination and to the taking of photographs must be obtained. Following this, a history of the attack must be taken, including the date, time and place, the nature of the attack, and whether drugs or alcohol were involved. It should be ascertained if the victim has bathed or washed after the attack, which may lead to crucial evidence against the perpetrator being lost.
- A thorough medical, gynaecological and obstetric history should also be taken and the state of the clothing recorded.
- This should be followed by a complete top to toe inspection, noting any signs of injury. Details of the nature and location of the injuries should be documented, noting bruising or petechiae, ligature marks, bite marks and defence wounds.
- Forensic samples should be obtained and meticulously labelled. The method by which these samples are obtained, the times when vaginal swabs, blood and urine samples are taken must also be recorded. The victim should be made to stand on a piece of paper while undressing, and any debris which falls must be collected. The piece of paper can be folded and retained. Swabs from the skin and all orifices, including mouth, low and high vaginal, endocervical and anal swabs must be taken. A detailed vaginal and anal examination must be done to look for signs of injury and to collect semen samples. Hair, blood and urine samples should be obtained.
- Thorough sexually transmitted disease screening should be done about a week later, and HIV testing recommended after counselling.
- The emergency postcoital contraception should be offered if deemed necessary.
- A trained rape counsellor should take over the counselling of the woman.

Q141. An 18-year-old girl complains of a vaginal discharge and has triple swabs taken which are reported positive for *Chlamydia*. Critically appraise how you will counsel and treat the girl.

A141.

- *Chlamydia* is the most frequent organism found in the genital tract of the young sexually active population and should be treated immediately in view of the havoc it can wreak on the reproductive potential of the woman.
- The girl should be instantly referred to the genitourinary medicine (GUM) clinic, there preferably being a means of automatic referral once a positive culture has been identified by the microbiology laboratories. This will ensure adequate treatment and follow-up, as well as contact tracing and the notification and treatment of all sexual partners.
- Before treatment, the girl should be provided with verbal and written information about the infection and its possible complications.
- *Chlamydia* is one of the foremost causes of tubal factor infertility, resulting in 8% of infertility after one episode, and 20% and 40% after two and three episodes of the infection, respectively. It is also responsible for an increase in the rate of ectopic pregnancy in these women. Thus, the importance of compliance to treatment of both the girl and her sexual partners needs to be stressed.
- Treatment needs to be started with tetracyclines, either doxycycline or minocycline for a minimum duration of a week to 10 days. They are contraindicated in patients with renal failure and in pregnant women. In these cases, erythromycin can be used safely and effectively.
- In women where non-compliance is a real risk, a single dose of 1 g azithromycin can be used.
- Screening for other sexually transmitted infections should be carried out with consent, including testing for gonorrhoea and HIV. Other sexually transmitted diseases may often coexist with *Chlamydia* and need to be treated separately.
- The patient should be warned against high risk sexual behaviour and strongly recommended the use of barrier contraception to prevent future episodes.

Chapter 11
Gynaecological oncology

Chapter 11: **Questions**

Answers are on pp. 168–178

Q142. A routine smear on a 35-year-old woman taken by her GP is reported as moderately dyskaryotic. It turns out that she is 8 weeks pregnant. The GP writes to you for advice. Justify the advice you will impart and your management plan.

Q143. A 68-year-old lady is referred to your gynaecology clinic with a history of vulval pruritis. On local examination she is found to have thinning and atrophy of the vulval skin with patchy white areas and fusion of the labia. How will you reach a diagnosis and institute treatment?

Q144. Debate the need for gynaecology–oncology centres.

Q145. A woman is admitted to the gynaecology ward with vaginal bleeding and a positive pregnancy test. A subsequent ultrasound scan reveals a complete molar pregnancy. Justify your management and counselling.

Q146. A recent smear report on a 40-year-old patient has revealed the presence of atypical glandular cells suggestive of cervical intraepithelial glandular neoplasia. Justify your management.

Q147. A woman who is being investigated for postmenopausal bleeding undergoes a hysteroscopy and endometrial sampling which reveals endometrial carcinoma. How will you go about managing the case?

Q148. A 63-year-old woman is referred by her GP for a suspicious vulval lesion. A subsequent biopsy reveals squamous carcinoma. Critically appraise the principles of management of this case.

Q149. Critically appraise the management of non-epithelial ovarian cancers.

Q150. A 72-year-old woman who has undergone chemotherapy for widespread metastatic ovarian cancer is admitted to hospital with symptoms of pain, vomiting and constipation. Critically appraise the principles of palliative therapy.

Q151. Critically appraise the side-effects of chemotherapeutic agents used for the treatment of epithelial ovarian cancers and how best to minimize them.

Q152. A case of postmenopausal bleeding is investigated and is found to be papillary serous carcinoma of the endometrium, with involvement of the outer half of the myometrium. Critically appraise the optimal treatment for the tumour.

Q153. Critically appraise the management of endometrial hyperplasia.

Q154. A 35-year-old woman is seen in the colposcopy clinic for a cytological abnormality on a cervical smear. Colposcopic examination reveals a low grade abnormality and a decision for conservative management is taken. Critically appraise how you will plan follow-up of the case.

Chapter 11: **Answers**

Q142. A routine smear on a 35-year-old woman taken by her GP is reported as moderately dyskaryotic. It turns out that she is 8 weeks pregnant. The GP writes to you for advice. Justify the advice you will impart and your management plan.

A142.

- Recommendations for referral for abnormal smears in pregnancy are the same as for non-pregnant women. Therefore, those with moderately dyskaryotic smears or worse should be referred for colposcopy and those with lesser abnormalities should undergo a repeat smear in 6 months. It is important to bear in mind the poorer quality of smears and the much larger transformation zone in pregnant women.
- Colposcopic examination should be carried out after reassuring the woman that the procedure does not harm the fetus or cause miscarriage. As colposcopy in pregnancy is technically difficult, it should be performed by a person experienced in the procedure.
- Time should be taken to visualize the whole of the transformation zone carefully as a small field of CIN may be present within much wider areas of metaplasia. It is important not to over-diagnose CIN because of the increased vascularity of the cervix.
- Treatment of CIN is not indicated in pregnancy and thus there is no justification in taking directed biopsies. This is because there is an increased risk of haemorrhage in pregnancy, added to which there is more of a chance of an unsatisfactory sample and they are unreliable in diagnosing invasive disease.
- If invasive disease is suspected, a large cervical wedge biopsy should be done under a general anaesthetic by an experienced person.
- If colposcopy suggests no more than CIN I, a repeat assessment is done 3 months after delivery.
- If a colposcopic examination suggests CIN II or III, which is likely in this case due to the moderately dyskaryotic smear, colposcopy should be repeated at the end of the second trimester.
- Postnatal examination may be made difficult due to the hypo-oestrogenic condition of the vagina and cervix and a 6-week course of local oestrogen therapy may be helpful.

Q143. A 68-year-old lady is referred to your gynaecology clinic with a history of vulval pruritis. On local examination she is found to have thinning and atrophy of the vulval skin with patchy white areas and fusion of the labia. How will you reach a diagnosis and institute treatment?

A143.

- The most likely diagnosis in this case is that of lichen sclerosis, which is a condition associated with autoimmune disorders. Clinically, there may be vulval pain and dyspareunia in addition to pruritis.
- The typical appearance of lichen sclerosis is that of irregular flat-topped white papules, which become atrophic and coalesce, leading to fusion of the labia and sometimes clitoral adhesions and shrinkage of the introitus. There may be fissuring of the skin due to severe hyperkeratosis.
- Although a benign condition, it may be found adjacent to vulval cancers in up to 32% of cases, and may progress to vulval cancer in 3–5% of cases. It is thus important to biopsy any suspicious areas before commencing treatment.
- Treatment is with the topical application of a potent steroid such as clobetasone propionate (Dermovate) for a period of up to 12 weeks. Once the symptoms have subsided, maintenance treatment can be with a less potent steroid with antifungal such as Trimovate.
- Testosterone cream is ineffective in improving the condition and should not be used.
- Surgical excision of these areas is not recommended as recurrences are common following excision or vulvectomy. Surgery to divide the adherent labia is unlikely to be of benefit unless topical steroids are used before and afterwards.
- It is important to keep these women under surveillance because of the risk of developing vulval cancer.

Q144. Debate the need for gynaecology–oncology centres.

A144.

- The concept of gynaecology–oncology centres (GOC) was introduced in response to the Calman–Hine report from the Department of Health which recommended the setting up of cancer centres where expert care could be delivered to patients with improved psychosocial support. The GOC is a tight organizational unit with expert groups of surgical oncologists as well as clinical and medical oncologists working together in a multidisciplinary team which also comprises pathologists, radiologists, clinical nurse specialists, physiotherapists, dietitians, lymphoedema specialists and radiation therapists. They are all fully trained and accredited in cancer care.
- There is evidence to prove that higher survival rates ensue when gynaecological cancers such as ovarian and cervical cancers and procedures such as pelvic exanteration are carried out by specialist gynaecological

oncologists as compared to general gynaecologists or general surgeons. As the number of patients seen and treated in GOCs are higher, surgeons can develop and maintain the necessary skills and expertise in order to ensure better results.

- Treatment and follow-up at multidisciplinary centres such as GOCs are an independent predictor of survival, reducing the risk of death by 40%.
- Concentration of care of gynaecological cancers in centralized units ensures recruitment of larger numbers of patients to national and international trials, thus enabling vital research and development.
- These specialized centres can provide much needed psychological and emotional support by trained nurse specialists and Macmillan nurses. This is a very important role in the care of these patients and their families.
- These centres should audit their results and ensure high quality outcome data, comparable with international best practice. This ensures optimal results.
- These centres ensure adequate training to those wishing to subspecialize in gynaecological oncology.

Q145. A woman is admitted to the gynaecology ward with vaginal bleeding and a positive pregnancy test. A subsequent ultrasound scan reveals a complete molar pregnancy. Justify your management and counselling.

A145.

- A complete hydatidiform mole is an abnormal conceptus without an embryo and with gross hydropic swelling of the placental villi. The major long-term risk is the development of either invasive mole or choriocarcinoma. The risk of developing choriocarcinoma after a complete hydatidiform mole is 2–3%.
- Suction evacuation is the method of choice for evacuation of complete molar pregnancies.
- Medical termination, including cervical preparation prior to suction evacuation should be avoided where possible because of the increased need for chemotherapy in cases of medical terminations.
- Oxytocic agents should be avoided until evacuation has been completed because of the risk of dissemination of trophoblastic tissue into the circulation. If bleeding is severe prior to complete evacuation, a single dose of ergometrine may be used if unavoidable as this is less likely to produce embolization of trophoblast than the repeated contractions produced by oxytocin or prostaglandins.

- Mifepristone should be avoided for termination.
- Products of conception should be sent for histological diagnosis.
- All women with molar pregnancies should be registered and followed up by one of the screening centres for England, Scotland and Wales.
- There is no indication for the routine use of a second uterine evacuation, and if symptoms persist after the initial evacuation, consultation with the screening centre should be carried out prior to any further surgical intervention.
- Women should be advised not to conceive until they have had 6 months of normal hCG levels. After conclusion of any further pregnancy, further samples of urine and serum should be followed up to eliminate the risk of recurrence.
- Women should be reassured regarding future pregnancies, as the risk of recurrence is low (1 : 74).
- The combined oral contraceptive pill should be discouraged until hCG levels have been normal for at least 3 months as there is a higher risk of requiring chemotherapy.

Q146. A recent smear report on a 40-year-old patient has revealed the presence of atypical glandular cells suggestive of cervical intraepithelial glandular neoplasia. Justify your management.

A146.

- Cervical intraepithelial glandular neoplasia and its diagnosis and treatment present a challenge due to its lack of characteristic colposcopic findings and inaccessible endocervical location. Due to this reason, the possibility of adenocarcinoma *in situ* has to be ruled out. As there are no colposcopic features diagnostic of a glandular lesion, the colposcopy should be urgently carried out within 4 weeks of the receipt of referral because of the possibility of the presence of invasive cancer.
- Clinical and colposcopic assessment should be carried out to determine whether an invasive lesion is visible. If it is, a cone biopsy should be carried out. A cylindrical cone is recommended to include the transformation zone and extend at least 25 mm up the endocervical canal.
- Careful examination of the squamous transformation zone is recommended as in 50% of cases, there is coexistence of cervical intraepithelial neoplasia.
- If after excision of the lesion, the margins are not clear of CIGN a further cone biopsy or alternatively, a hysterectomy is recommended.
- Consideration should be given to the possibility of endometrial pathology and endometrial sampling should be done if indicated.

- Follow-up with cytology is essential and must include endocervical brush smears. If glandular abnormality persists, a further cone biopsy or hysterectomy is essential.
- If an invasive lesion is diagnosed on cone biopsy, a radical hysterectomy is indicated.

Q147. A woman who is being investigated for postmenopausal bleeding undergoes a hysteroscopy and endometrial sampling which reveals endometrial carcinoma. How will you go about managing the case?
A147.
- Endometrial cancer is a condition mostly associated with the postmenopausal age group. It is thus essential to ensure optimal fitness for treatment, whether surgery or radiotherapy, in order to optimize results and reduce morbidity.
- Basic investigations in the form of a chest X-ray, full blood count, urea and electrolytes and creatinine, and urine analysis should be carried out. MRI is useful in evaluating myometrial invasion, with a reported accuracy of 70–80%.
- The treatment of choice is a total abdominal hysterectomy and bilateral salpingo-oophorectomy.
- It is not clear whether lymph node sampling improves survival and thus until the results of the ongoing MRC (ASTEC) trial are revealed, removal of lymph nodes will be an individual clinical judgement depending on results of MRI, risk factors or obvious nodal involvement. The advantage of lymphadenectomy is to spare the women without nodal disease the side-effects of radiotherapy.
- Radiotherapy can prolong survival in women with advanced or recurrent disease, or when surgery is not appropriate.
- Adjuvant radiotherapy does not influence survival, but it reduces the incidence of pelvic recurrence.
- Chemotherapy or hormone therapy are not effective in endometrial cancer and are not recommended.

Q148. A 63-year-old woman is referred by her GP for a suspicious vulval lesion. A subsequent biopsy reveals squamous carcinoma. Critically appraise the principles of management of this case.
A148.
- The treatment of all vulval cancers should be undertaken in a specialist cancer centre under a multidisciplinary team. The patient should be made

aware of the concept of management planning and also of the potential outcomes.

- Baseline investigations should be carried out to determine the presence or absence of metastatic disease and to evaluate fitness for treatment, both surgical and non-surgical. These include a full blood count, biochemical profile, chest X-ray and electrocardiogram, cervical smear if this has not been done and imaging of the groins and pelvis to attempt preoperative detection of enlarged nodes. Sometimes, a fine-needle aspiration or biopsy of suspicious nodes is warranted.
- In early stage disease, wide radical local excision is done. The excision should encompass all areas of atypical epithelium and include a margin of at least 1 cm of normal epithelium. Coexisting lichen sclerosis or vulval intraepithelial neoplasia may need to be biopsied to exclude invasion.
- A superficial and deep inguinofemoral node dissection is recommended for groin nodes. This should be done in all squamous cancers other than stage Ia. If excision of the primary vulval tumour does not impinge on a midline structure then only the ipsilateral groin need initially be resected. If positive nodes are found then the other groin will need dissection.
- In centrally located tumours, wide local excision with bilateral lymphadenectomy via a triple incision technique is the procedure of choice.
- The management of large lesions depends upon a multimodality approach. Preoperative radiotherapy with or without concurrent chemotherapy can allow for sphincter conservation at the time of radical excision.

Q149. Critically appraise the management of non-epithelial ovarian cancers.

A149.

- Non-epithelial ovarian cancers constitute approximately 10% of all ovarian cancers. They mainly constitute germ cell tumours and sex cord–stromal tumours. The former are derived from the primitive germ cells of the primitive gonads, occurring mainly in young women in their early twenties. The latter constitute 7% of ovarian tumours, and a majority (70%) are made up of granulosa and theca cell tumours.
- Germ cell tumours mainly consist of dysgerminomas (48%) followed by endodermal sinus tumours (20%). Surgical management involves decisions concerning a conservative approach with future childbearing balanced against the probability of recurrence. Surgery is reserved for stage Ia tumours with cisplatin-based chemotherapy for all other stages. Serum

tumour markers like α-fetoprotein, human chorionic gonadotrophin, lactate dehydrogenase and inhibin may be useful in diagnosis and follow-up.

- Most granulosa cell tumours are unilateral and may produce sex steroids, resulting in postmenopausal bleeding in older women or sexual precocity in prepubertal girls. They may be bilateral in 5% of cases. Unilateral oophorectomy is indicated only in young women with stage I disease. Stage II–IV tumours need adjuvant chemotherapy. Prognosis is good with 5-year survival rates of 80%, but long-term follow-up is essential due to the propensity for late recurrences.

- The most common adjuvant chemotherapeutic drugs are VAC (vincristine, D-actinomycin, cyclophosphamide), VBP (vinblastine, bleomycin, cisplatin), and BEP (bleomycin, etoposide, cisplatin).

Q150. A 72-year-old woman who has undergone chemotherapy for widespread metastatic ovarian cancer is admitted to hospital with symptoms of pain, vomiting and constipation. Critically appraise the principles of palliative therapy.

A150.

- In the case of terminal malignancy, it is imperative to ensure freedom from pain and other troublesome symptoms which are a great part of the condition. A patient free of these symptoms is better placed to face her illness. These symptoms can be totally controlled in up to 95% of patients, and if they are not, specialist advice should be sought.

- The concept of the World Health Organization analgesic ladder where non-opioid analgesics and adjuvants are used for mild pain, progressing successively to a combination of opioids and non-opioids along with adjuvant analgesics for more severe pain should be used. Non-steroidal anti-inflammatory drugs can be given in the form of tablets, suspension, or rectal suppositories, bearing in mind that asthma, fluid retention and renal functions can all be worsened by their use. Misoprostol or H_2-antagonists should be given to those at risk of gastroduodenal ulceration or those on steroids.

- Opioids in the form of morphine are used to gain control of the pain with immediate release preparations, followed by modified release preparations for maintenance. In case this is not tolerated fentanyl in the form of transdermal patches can be used.

- Neuropathic pain due to damage to the nervous system is relieved by adjuvant analgesics such as tricyclic antidepressants, anticonvulsants and corticosteroids.

- Analgesics as well as antiemetics can be combined and administered subcutaneously via syringe drivers.
- In case of difficulty in controlling pain without excessive side-effects, the epidural or spinal route can be used for opiate delivery.
- The cause of nausea and vomiting should be addressed. This includes changing or stopping drugs which cause them. Anticholinergic drugs should be avoided in gastric stasis. Abnormal biochemistry, especially hypercalcaemia should be corrected. Raised intracranial pressure should be treated with steroids.
- In the case of constipation, bowel obstruction should first be ruled out. Rectal stimulants in the form of glycerine suppositories or softeners in the form of enemas are used to relieve constipation. Hyoscine and octreotide are used to relieve intestinal colic and reduce secretions.
- The use of steroids should be considered. These can be used via the oral, subcutaneous, rectal, intravenous or intramuscular route. A maximum dose is initially started and then reduced as symptoms dictate.
- Regular reviews of pain management and other symptoms should be done by designated members of the team. Psychological support and counselling should be offered, with the use of benzodiazepines to relieve anxiety if necessary.

Q151. Critically appraise the side-effects of chemotherapeutic agents used for the treatment of epithelial ovarian cancers and how best to minimize them.

A151.
- Chemotherapy plays a major role in the management of epithelial ovarian cancers, used postoperatively to prolong clinical remission and survival, and for palliation in advanced or recurrent disease. All agents, however, have side-effects which need to be minimized in order to achieve maximum success and minimum discomfort for the patient.
- Platinum drugs are one of the most widely used drugs in ovarian cancer chemotherapy. Cisplatin causes severe nausea and vomiting and can cause permanent renal damage. Peripheral neuropathy and hearing loss may also occur. Adequate hydration must be ensured to prevent renal damage, with the use of 5-HT antagonists such as ondansetron to combat nausea and vomiting.
- Carboplatin causes less nausea and vomiting and does not possess renal toxicity. Intravenous hydration is thus not necessary though it can cause bone marrow suppression. Leucopaenia and thrombocytopaenia should be carefully monitored and treated.

- Alkylating agents such as cyclophosphamide, chlorambucil and melphelan can be given orally and cause mild nausea. They are toxic to the bone marrow and thus blood counts should be monitored and they should be given in intermittent courses.
- Paclitaxel (Taxol) is a new chemotherapeutic agent being increasingly used alone or in combination with platinum agents. Neutropenia is the principal toxicity and granulocyte colony-stimulating factor (G-CSF) is usually given to prevent this. Sensory neuropathy in the form of 'glove and stocking' paraesthesia is usually dose dependent and can be minimized by optimizing the dose given. Hypersensitivity reactions such as angioedema, respiratory distress, hypotension and urticaria may also be associated with Taxol and are minimized by a premed regimen of dexamethasone, diphenhydramine and cimetidine. Total body hair loss is the norm.
- Careful monitoring of full blood counts and differential count and platelets, renal and liver function tests needs to be undertaken. There is a risk of developing leukaemia with prolonged treatment and thus it should be limited to a maximum of 1 year.

Q152. A case of postmenopausal bleeding is investigated and is found to be papillary serous carcinoma of the endometrium, with involvement of the outer half of the myometrium. Critically appraise the optimal treatment for the tumour.

A152.

- Papillary serous carcinoma of the endometrium is a highly aggressive tumour, responsible (along with clear cell carcinoma of the endometrium) for about 50% of all relapses, with a 5-year survival of only 27%. It is important to treat these patients aggressively in order to prevent a recurrence.
- A thorough surgical staging and debulking procedure in the form of a total abdominal hysterectomy, bilateral salpingo-oophorectomy, pelvic and para-aortic lymphadenectomy, peritoneal washings, peritoneal biopsy and omentectomy should be undertaken.
- The most frequent extrapelvic sites of recurrence are the upper abdomen, lungs and liver.
- Adjuvant pelvic radiotherapy plus intracavitary radiotherapy is given in early stage disease. Pelvic radiotherapy or whole abdomen radiation is given in advanced stage disease.
- Systemic chemotherapy is usually administered with cisplatin, doxorubicin and cyclophosphamide (PAC), though increasingly, paclitaxel, alone

or in combination is being used. The use of chemotherapy as postoperative adjuvant treatment is still controversial.

Q153. Critically appraise the management of endometrial hyperplasia.
A153.

- Endometrial hyperplasia are a group of abnormalities of the endometrium representing premalignant lesions. Depending upon degree of cytological abnormality, they are classified as simple hyperplasia, complex hyperplasia, simple hyperplasia with atypia and complex hyperplasia with atypia. The diagnosis is made on endometrial biopsy, usually taken to investigate abnormal bleeding or discharge.
- The risk of progression of simple hyperplasia to carcinoma of the endometrium is very small. This increases to less than 5% in cases of complex hyperplasia, and up to 25–30% in complex hyperplasia with atypia.
- Predisposing factors for the development of hyperplasia include women with polycystic ovarian syndrome, those on unopposed oestrogens, tamoxifen therapy, obesity, anovulation and oestrogen-secreting tumours.
- Management of the condition will depend upon the type of hyperplasia, age of the woman as well as her desire to conserve her fertility. In the case of postmenopausal women with cytological atypia, especially with complex hyperplasia, there is a significant risk of progression to cancer and thus a total abdominal hysterectomy with bilateral salpingo-oophorectomy should be recommended. In women under 45 years, a hysterectomy alone can be advised, though this will depend upon the degree and extent of the atypical hyperplasia, and the risk of an invasive lesion being present.
- In women who wish to retain their fertility, or refuse to undergo a hysterectomy, high dose progestogens such as medroxyprogesterone acetate in a dose of 100 mg daily should be given for 6 months, with a repeat endometrial biopsy 3 months after cessation of treatment. Long-term close surveillance should continue, and the use of the levonorgestrel intrauterine system may be useful in controlling the hyperplasia.
- In the absence of atypia, in either simple or complex hyperplasia, management is symptomatic, usually with hormonal preparations to control irregular bleeding patterns.
- Though transvaginal ultrasound scanning is a useful tool in the evaluation of postmenopausal women with bleeding, this is not a good tool in the evaluation of perimenopausal or premenopausal women with symptoms. In postmenopausal women with an endometrial thickness less than 5 mm, the risk of endometrial abnormality is minimal.

Q154. A 35-year-old woman is seen in the colposcopy clinic for a cyto-logical abnormality on a cervical smear. Colposcopic examination reveals a low grade abnormality and a decision for conservative management is taken. Critically appraise how you will plan follow-up of the case.

A154.

- In women with low grade cytological and histological (CIN I/HPV associated changes) lesions, conservative management is an option because of the chance of regression of the abnormality and the risk of overtreatment were all such lesions to be excised. However, close surveillance is required in these cases.

- The decision for conservative management should be reached only after counselling of the woman and agreement for continued colposcopic and cytological surveillance. In case of any likelihood of non-compliance, treatment should be offered.

- Accurate colposcopic assessment and appropriate directed biopsies are necessary for women opting for conservative management. A deferred management strategy may be adopted only if the colposcopist is confident of the diagnosis.

- Colposcopy and cytology should be repeated at 6 monthly intervals. If the abnormality persists either colposcopically or cytologically (the upper limit being arbitrarily set at 24 months), treatment should be offered.

- If the lesion regresses, surveillance should continue until two consecutive smears are negative, at which point routine 3 yearly screening can recommence.